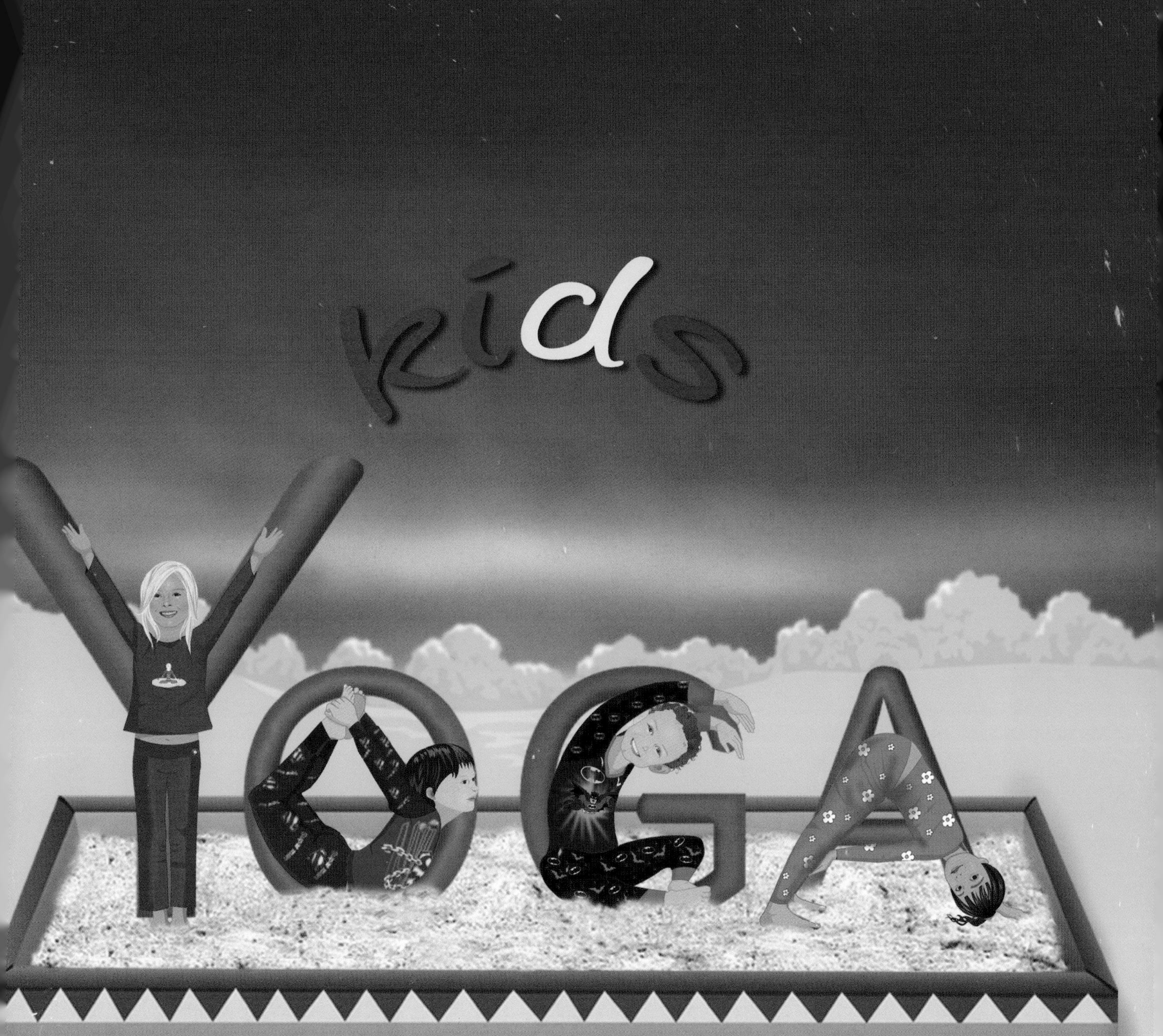

Author: Jeff Maier

Yoga started in India a long, long time ago
Yoga makes you feel good and helps you grow

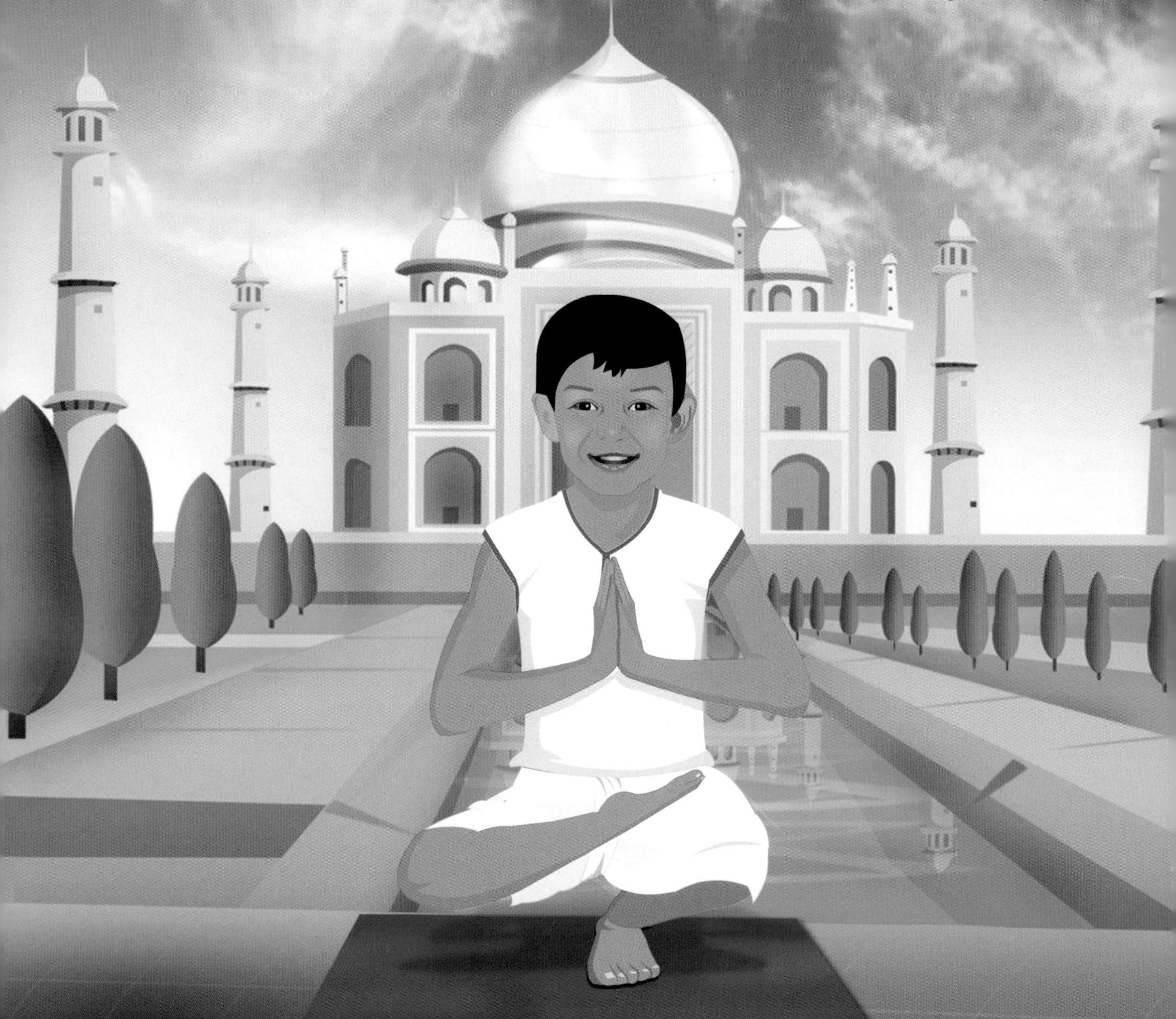

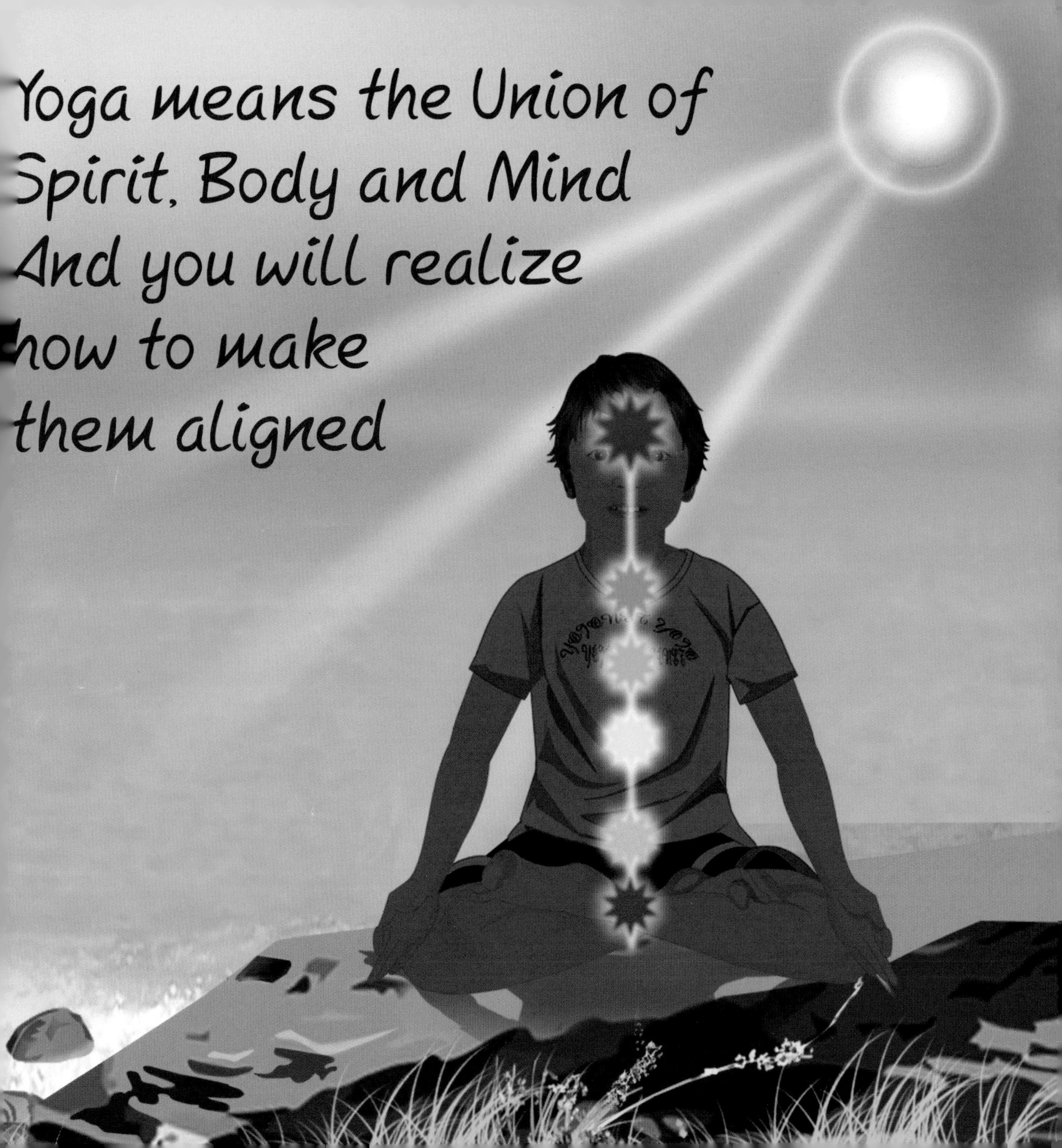
Yoga means the Union of
Spirit, Body and Mind
And you will realize
how to make
them aligned

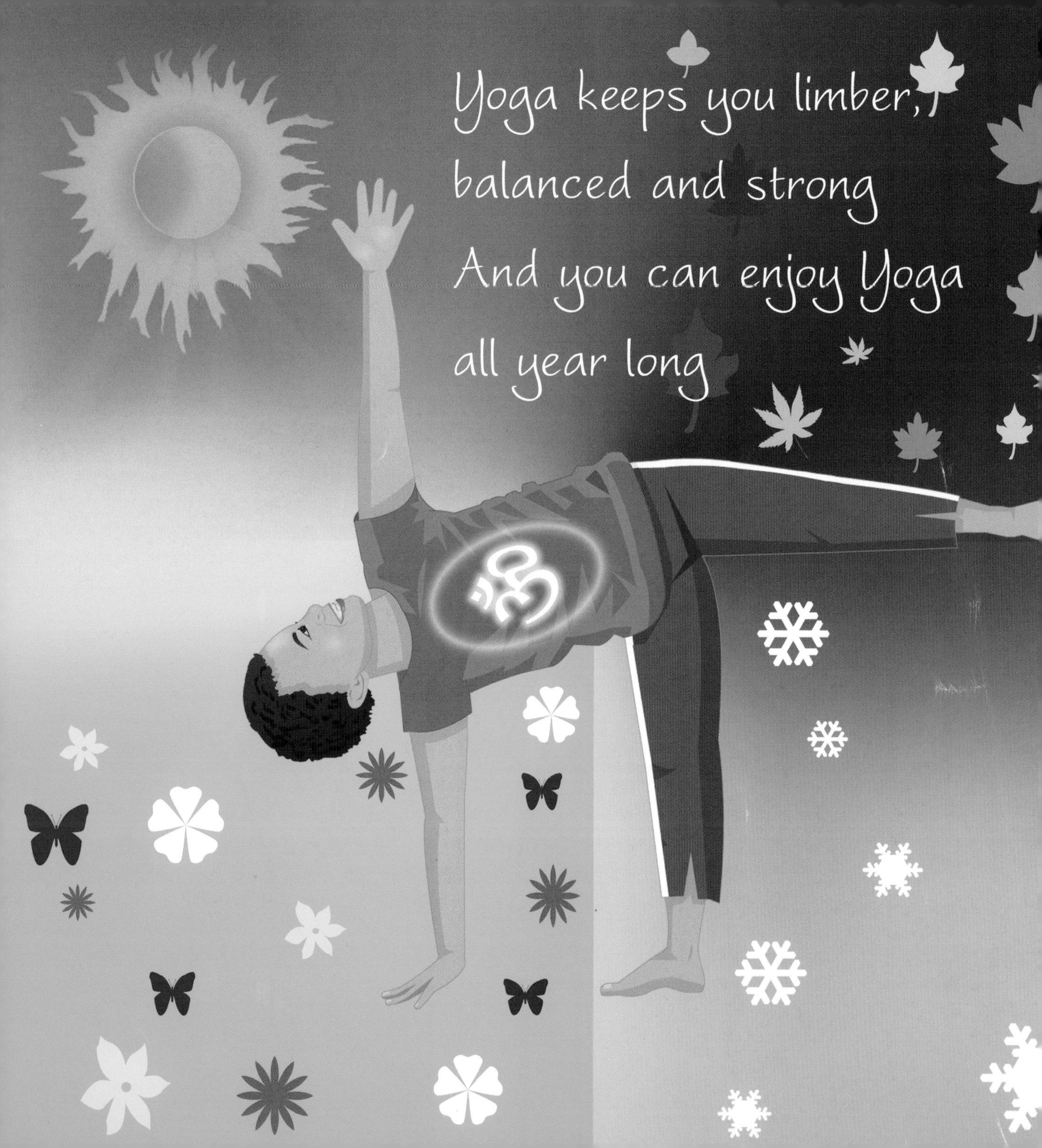
Yoga keeps you limber,
balanced and strong
And you can enjoy Yoga
all year long

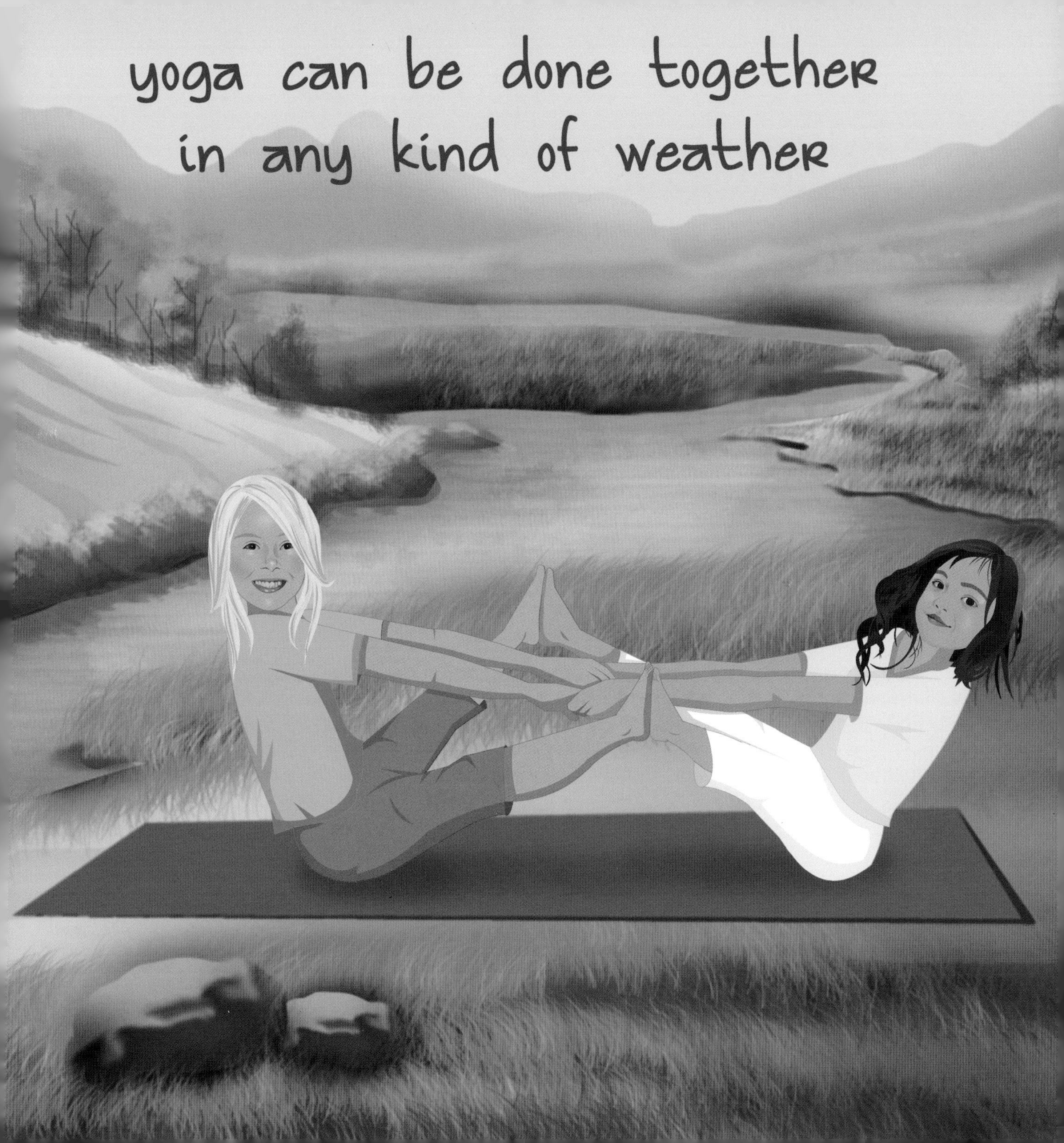
yoga can be done together
in any kind of weather

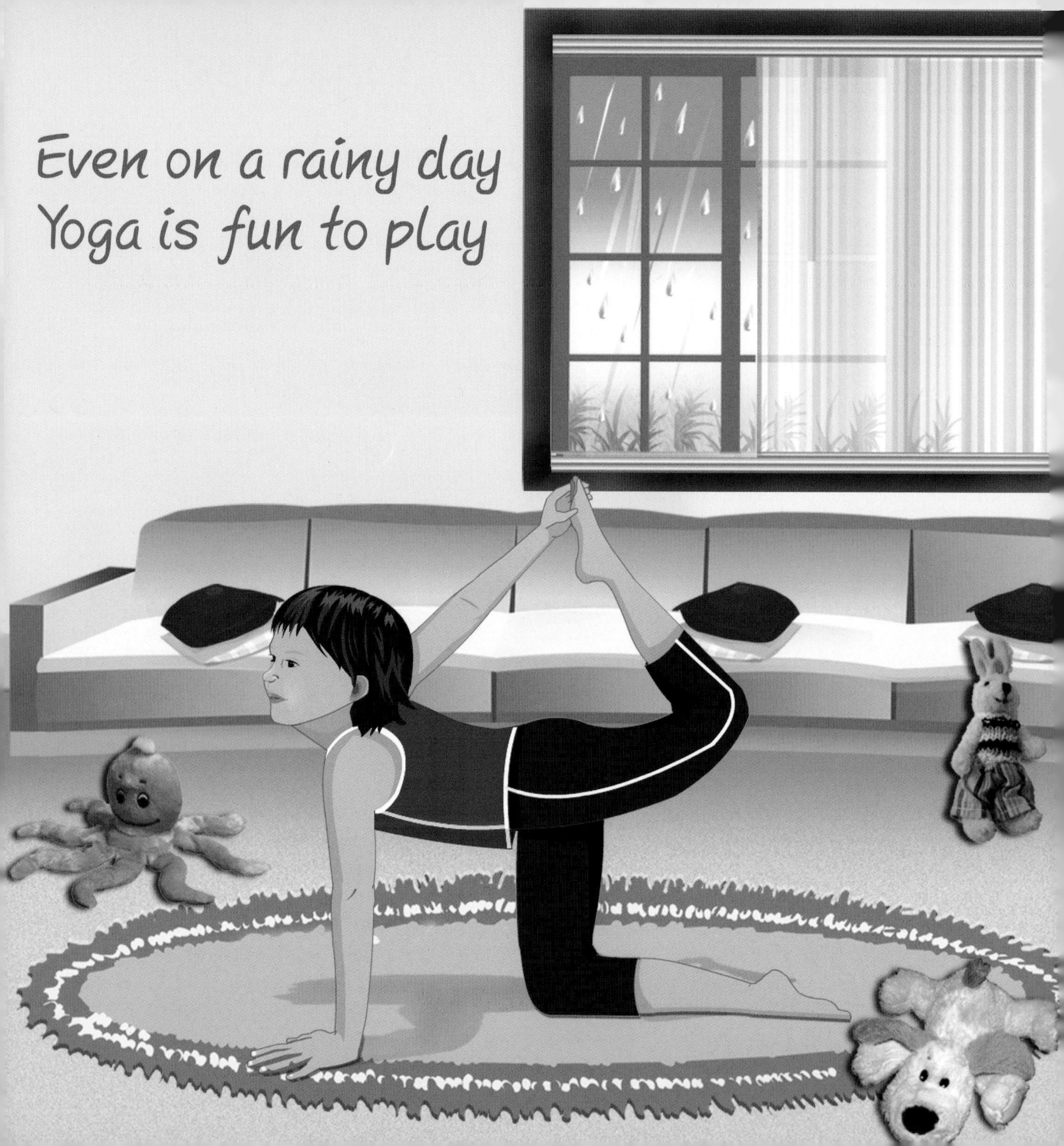
Even on a rainy day
Yoga is fun to play

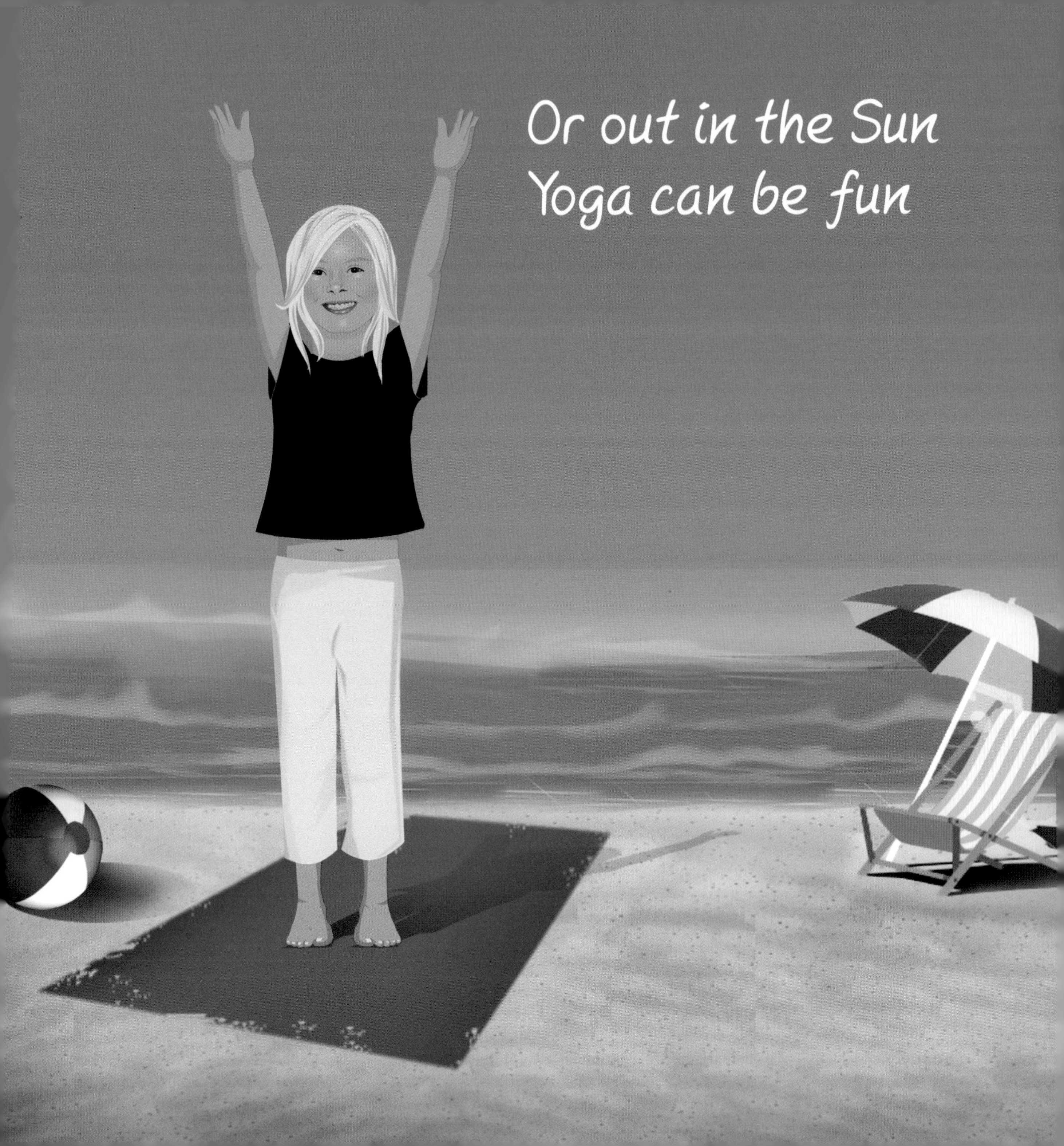

Or out in the Sun
Yoga can be fun

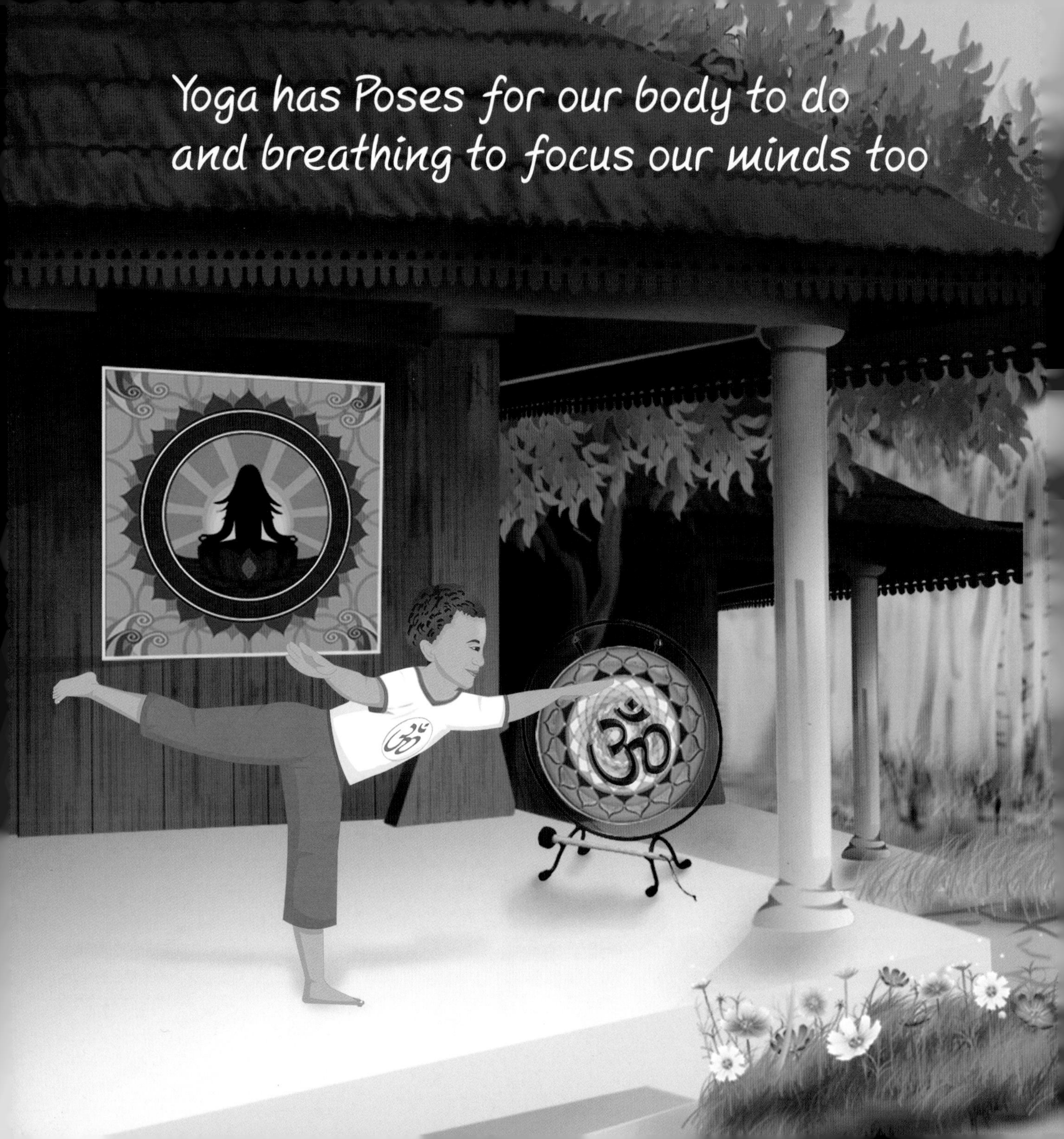

Yoga has Poses for our body to do
and breathing to focus our minds too

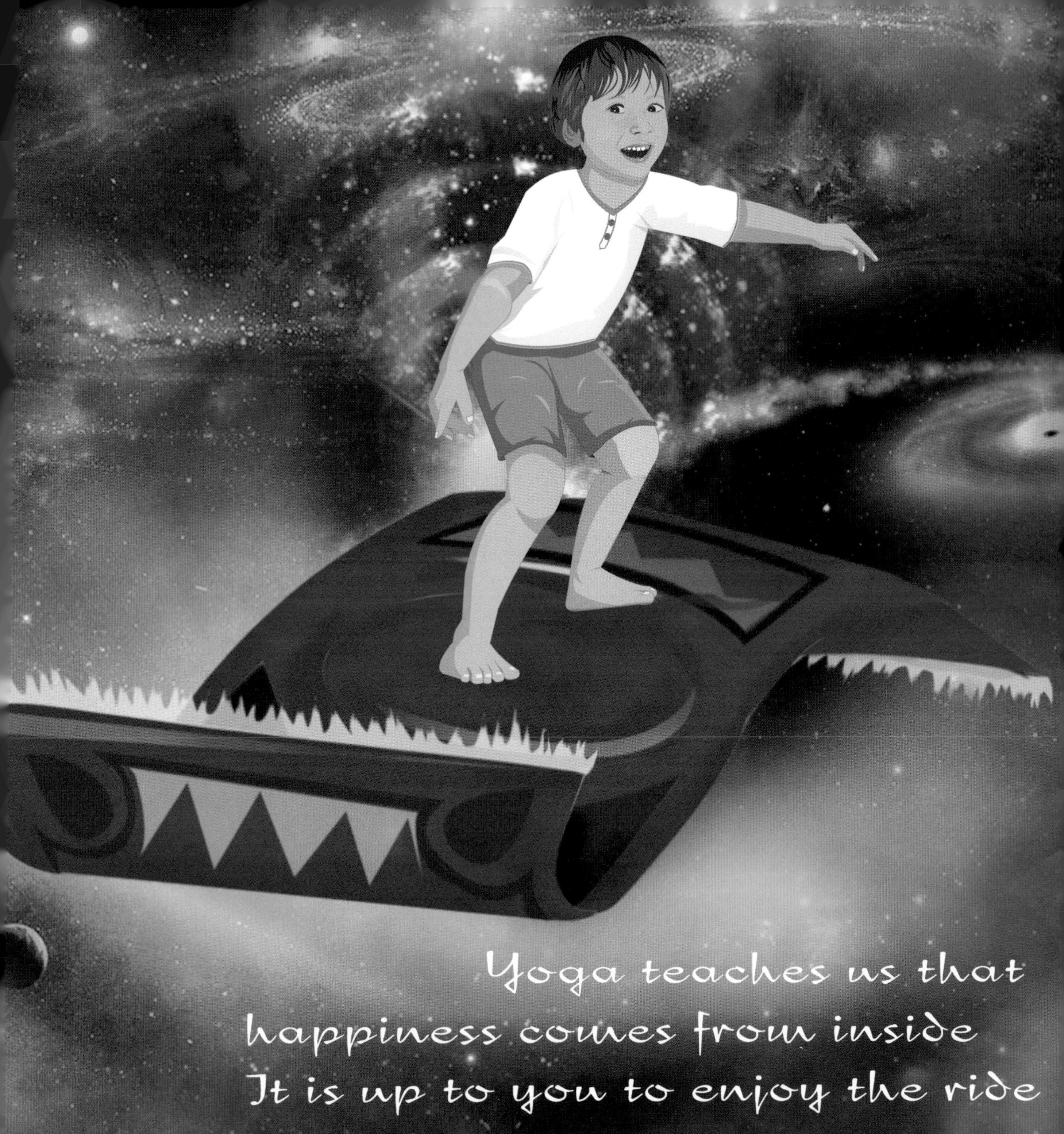
Yoga teaches us that
happiness comes from inside
It is up to you to enjoy the ride

Mountain pose is standing straight and strong
Can you do it?
How long?

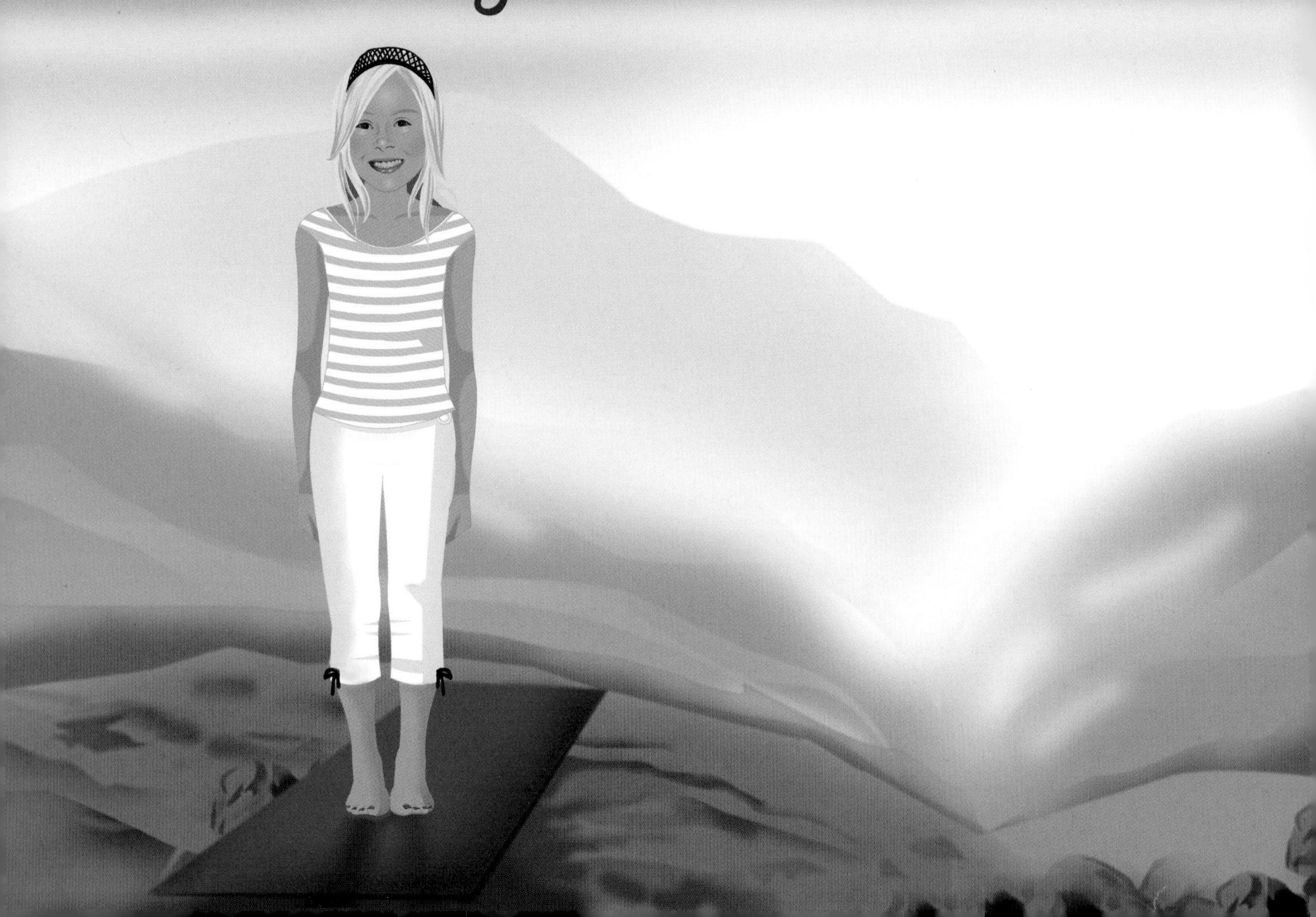

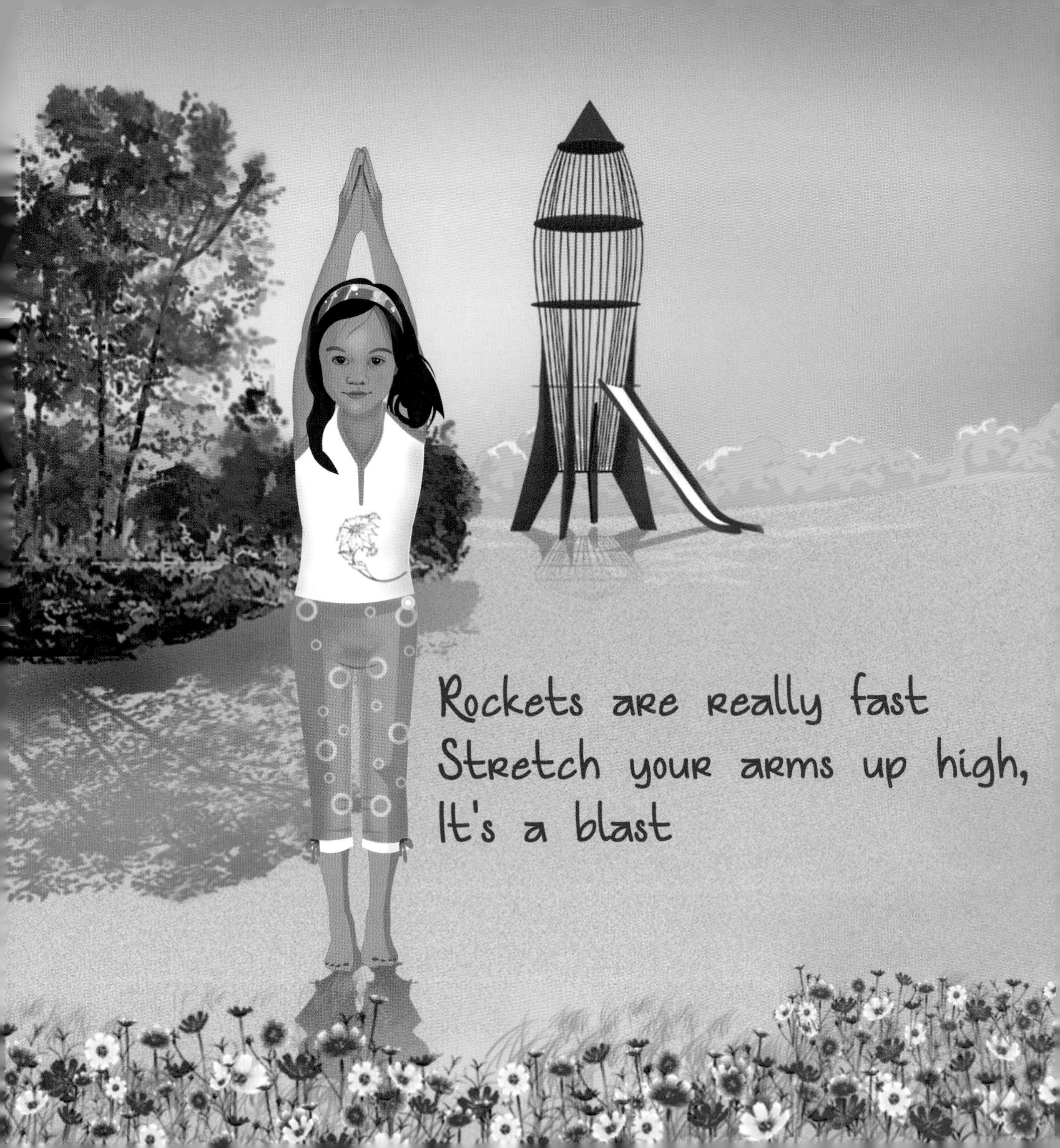

Rockets are really fast
Stretch your arms up high,
It's a blast

Half Moon is bending side to side
Making you feel good inside

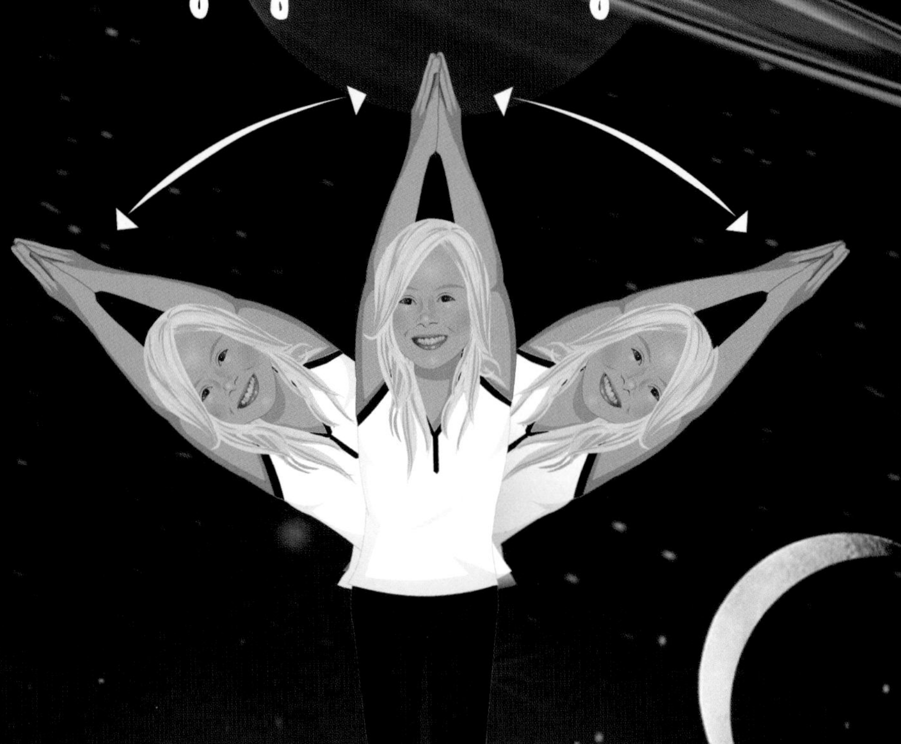

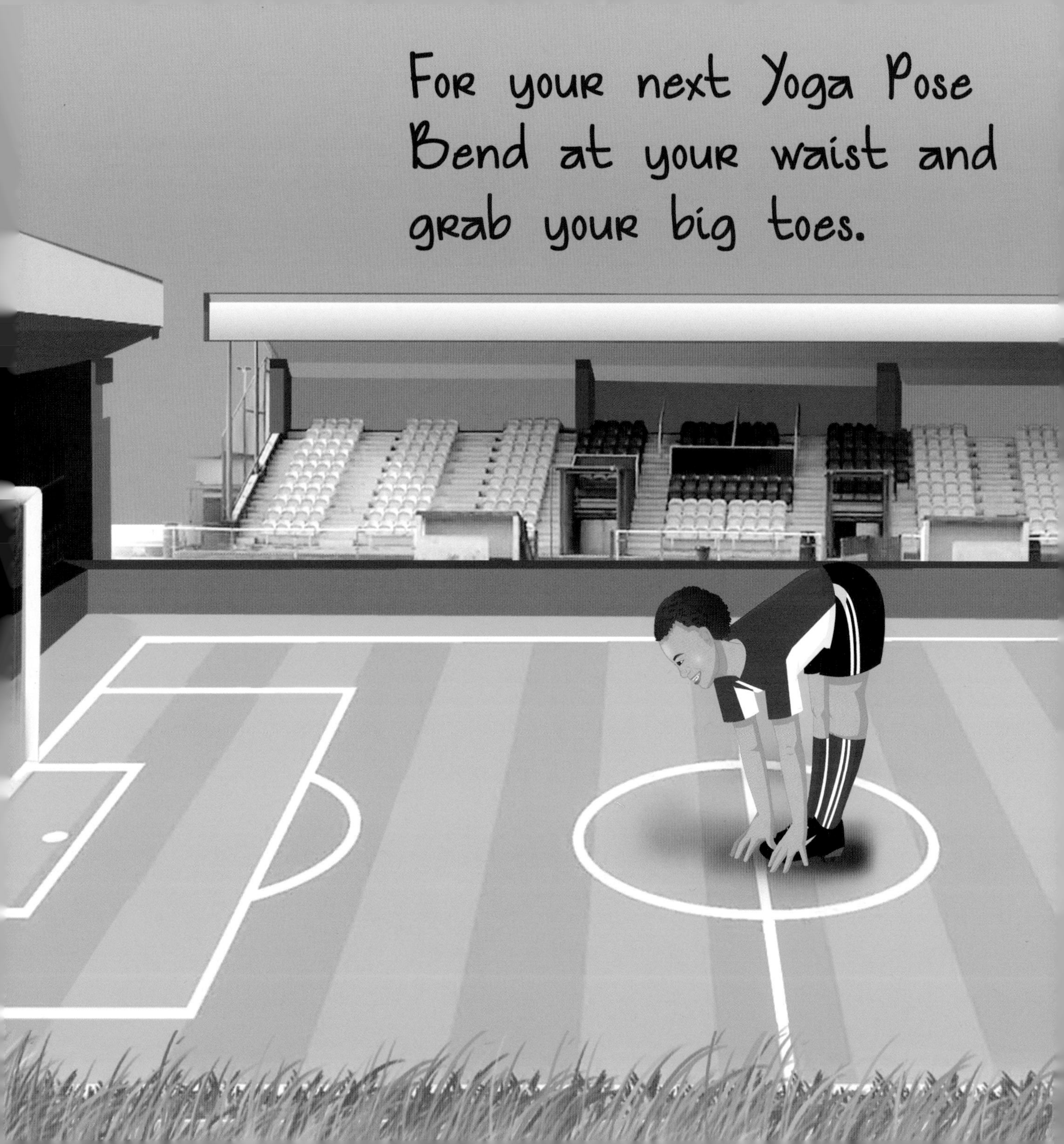

For your next Yoga Pose Bend at your waist and grab your big toes.

Be a Warrior for Peace Love and Jo

It is good for every girl and boy

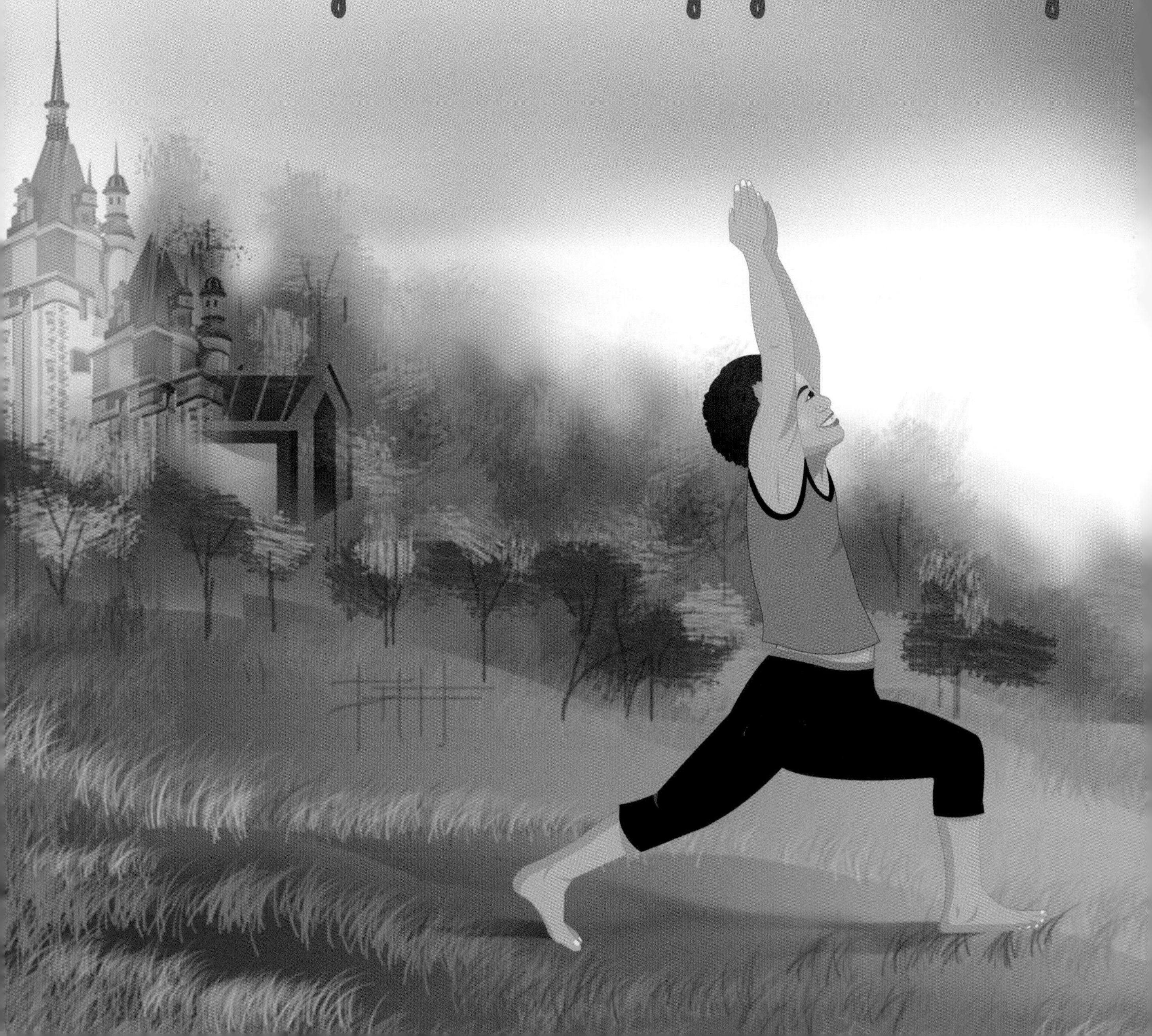

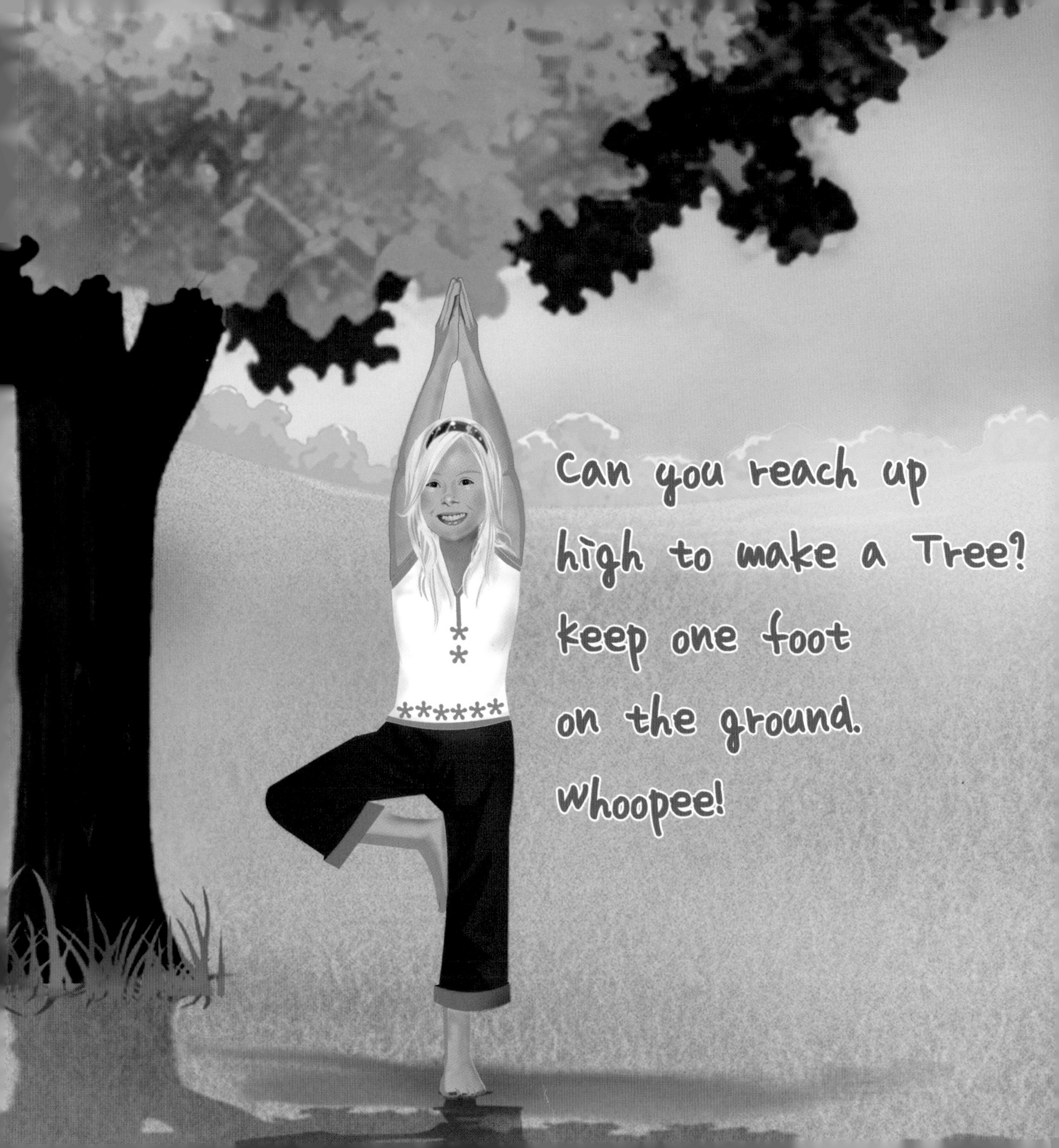
Can you reach up
high to make a Tree?
keep one foot
on the ground.
Whoopee!

Can you be a Frog?

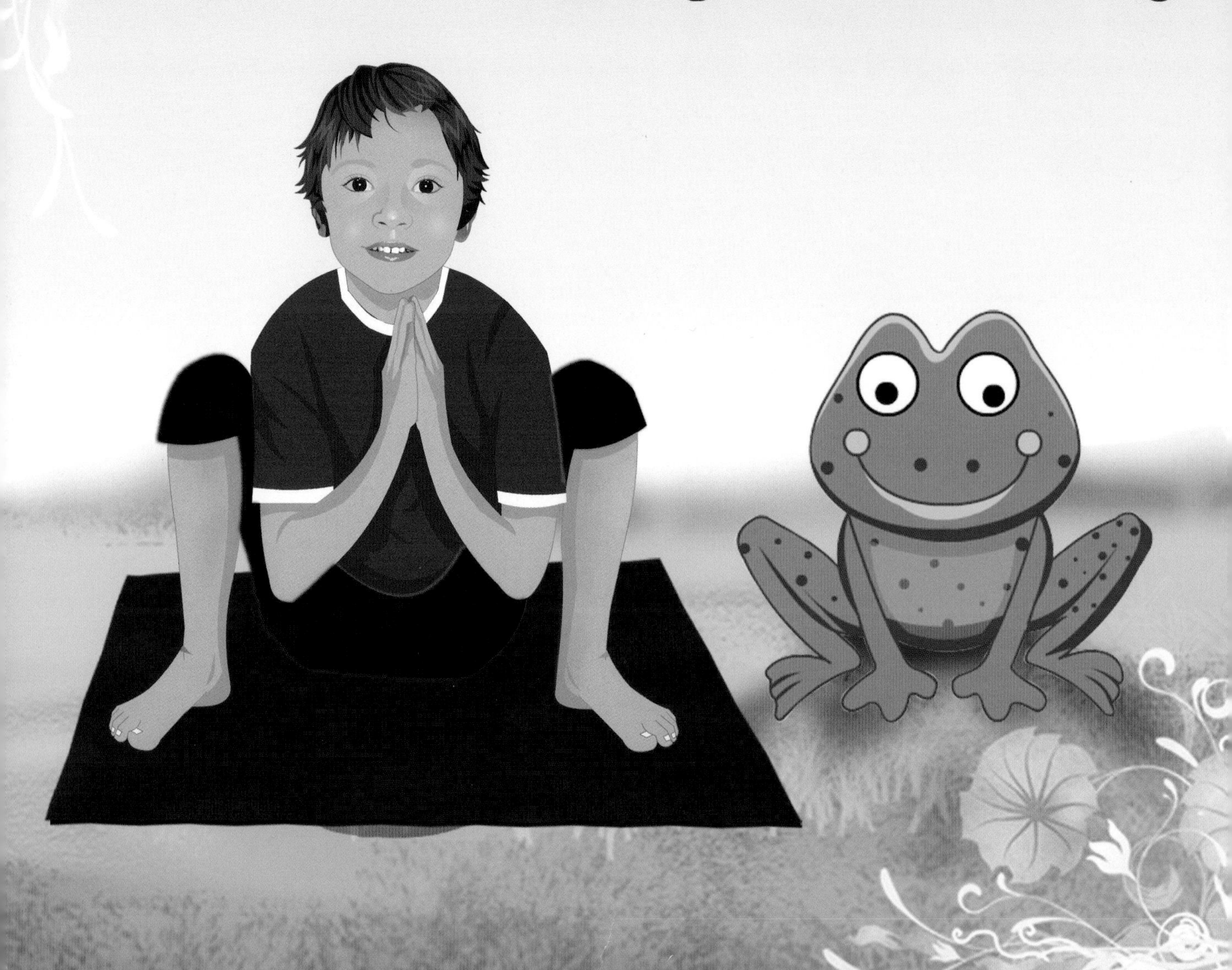

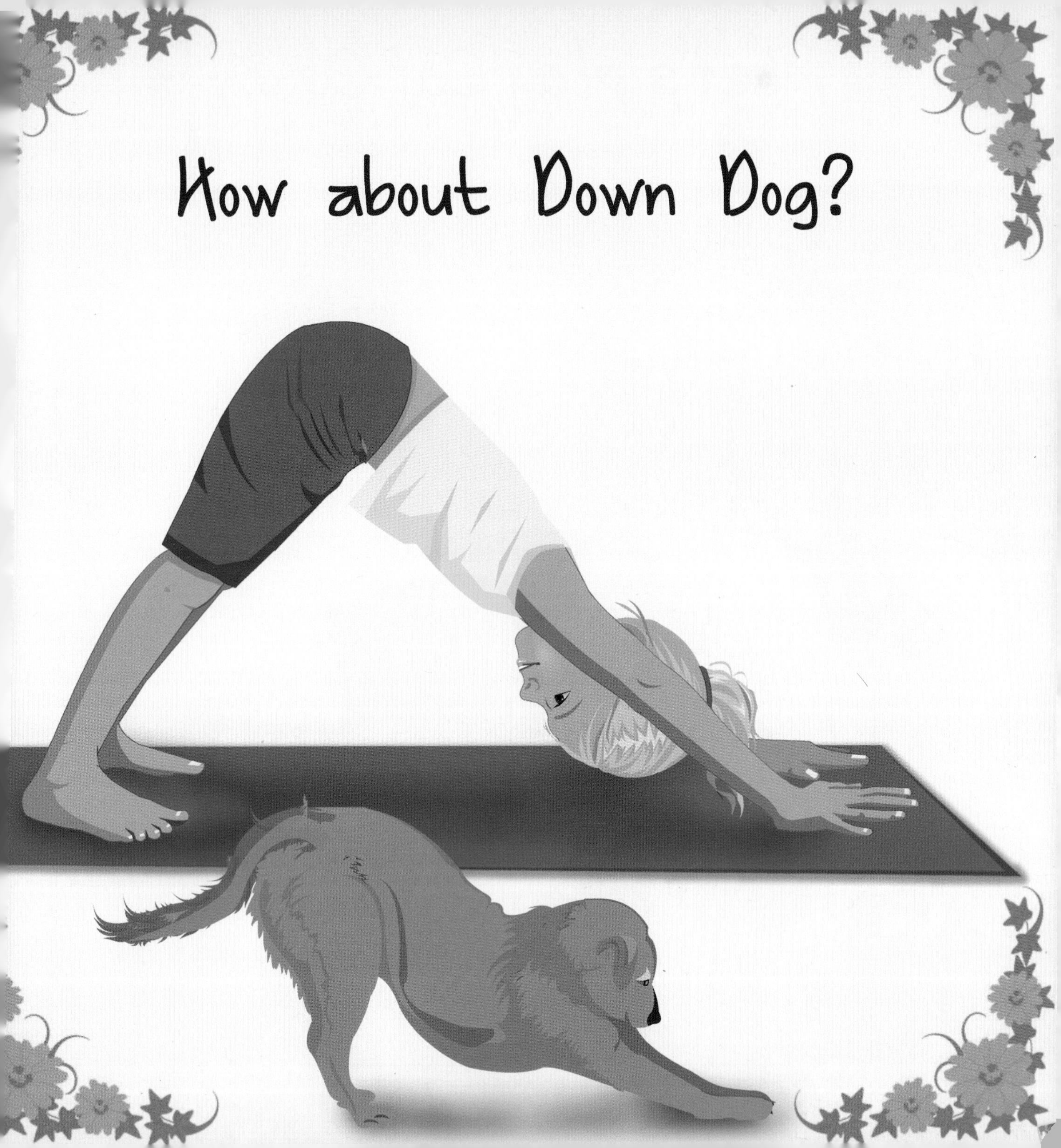
How about Down Dog?

Let's play Cat Cow...

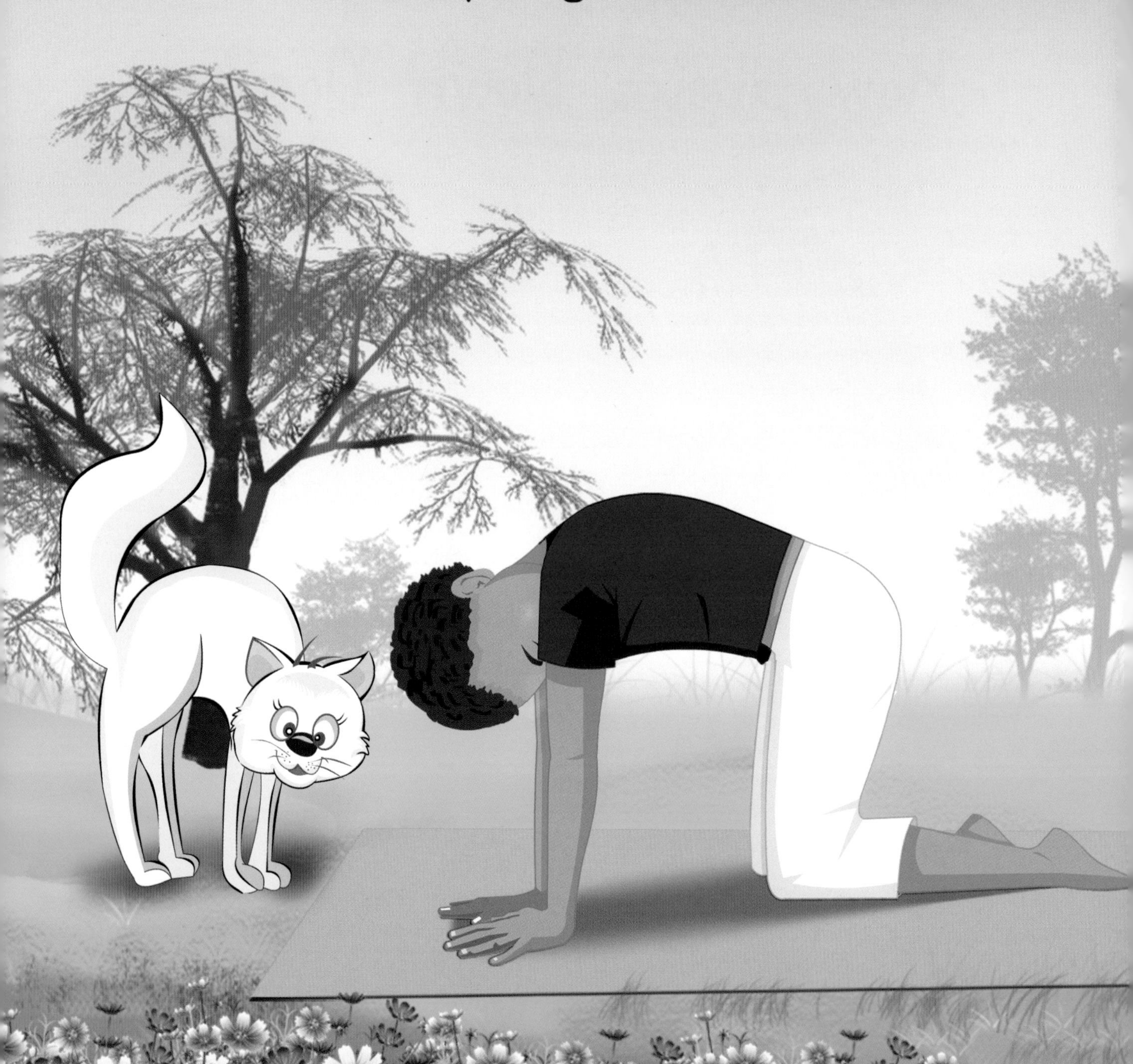

and say Moo and Meow !

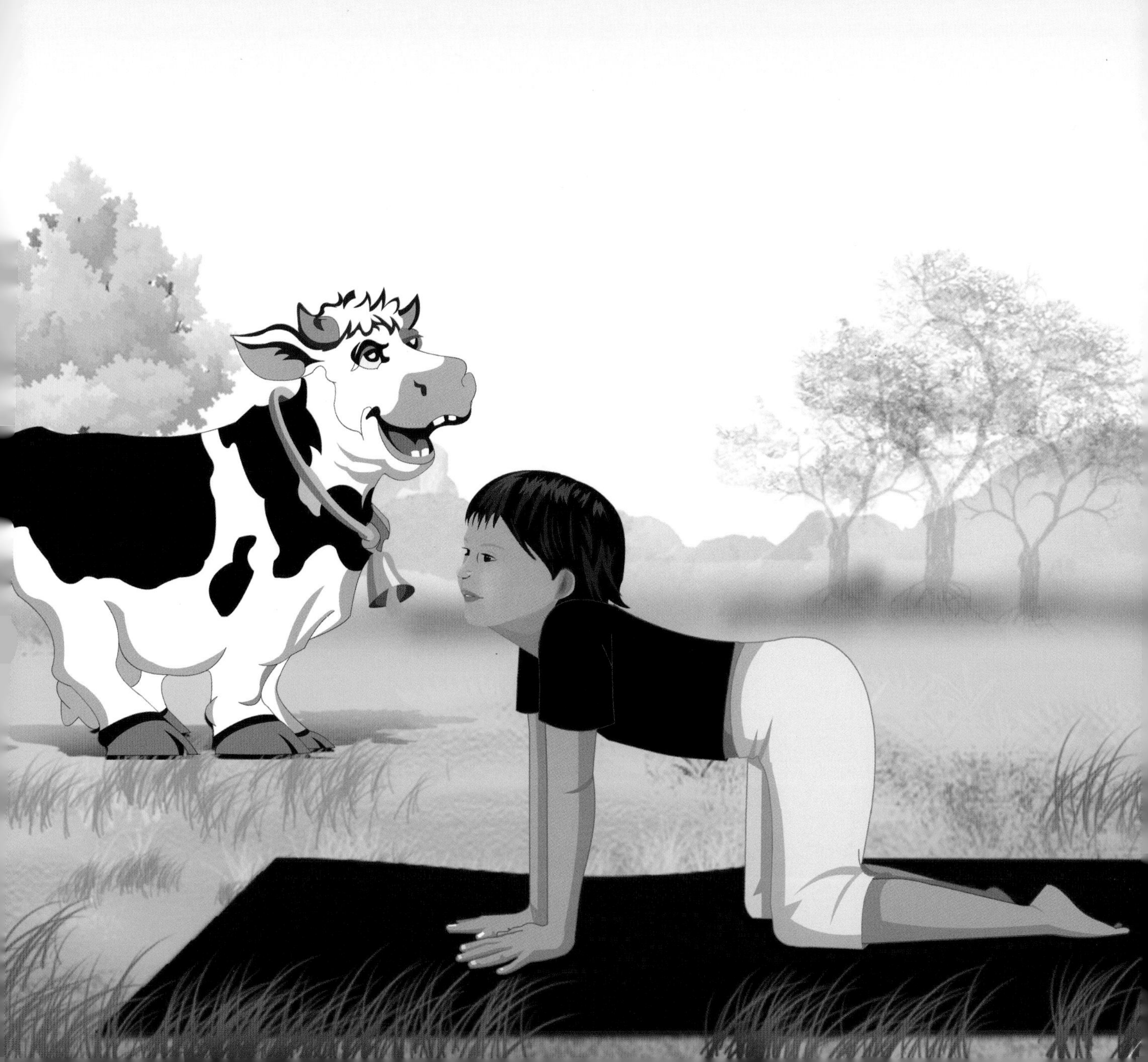

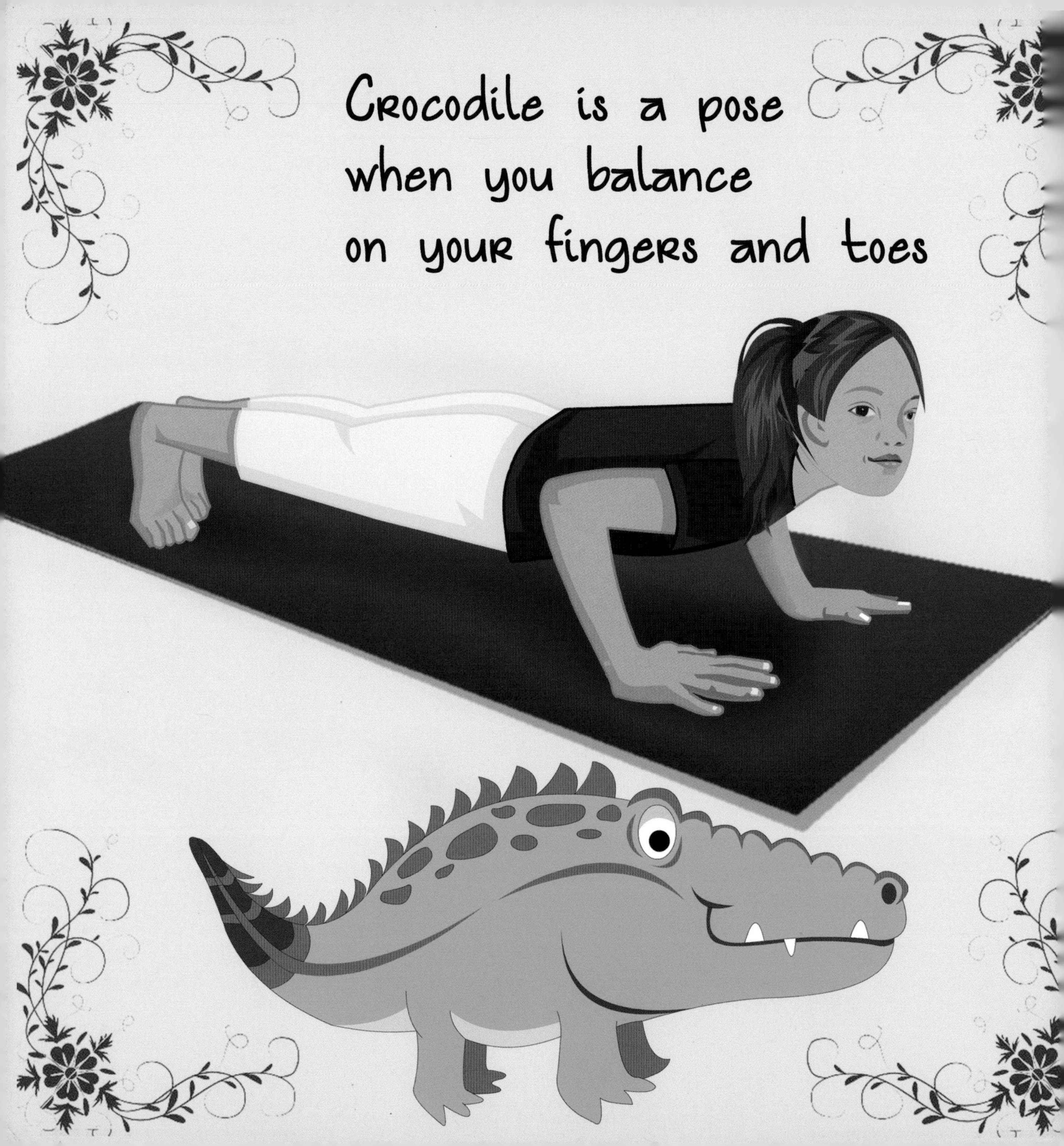
Crocodile is a pose
when you balance
on your fingers and toes

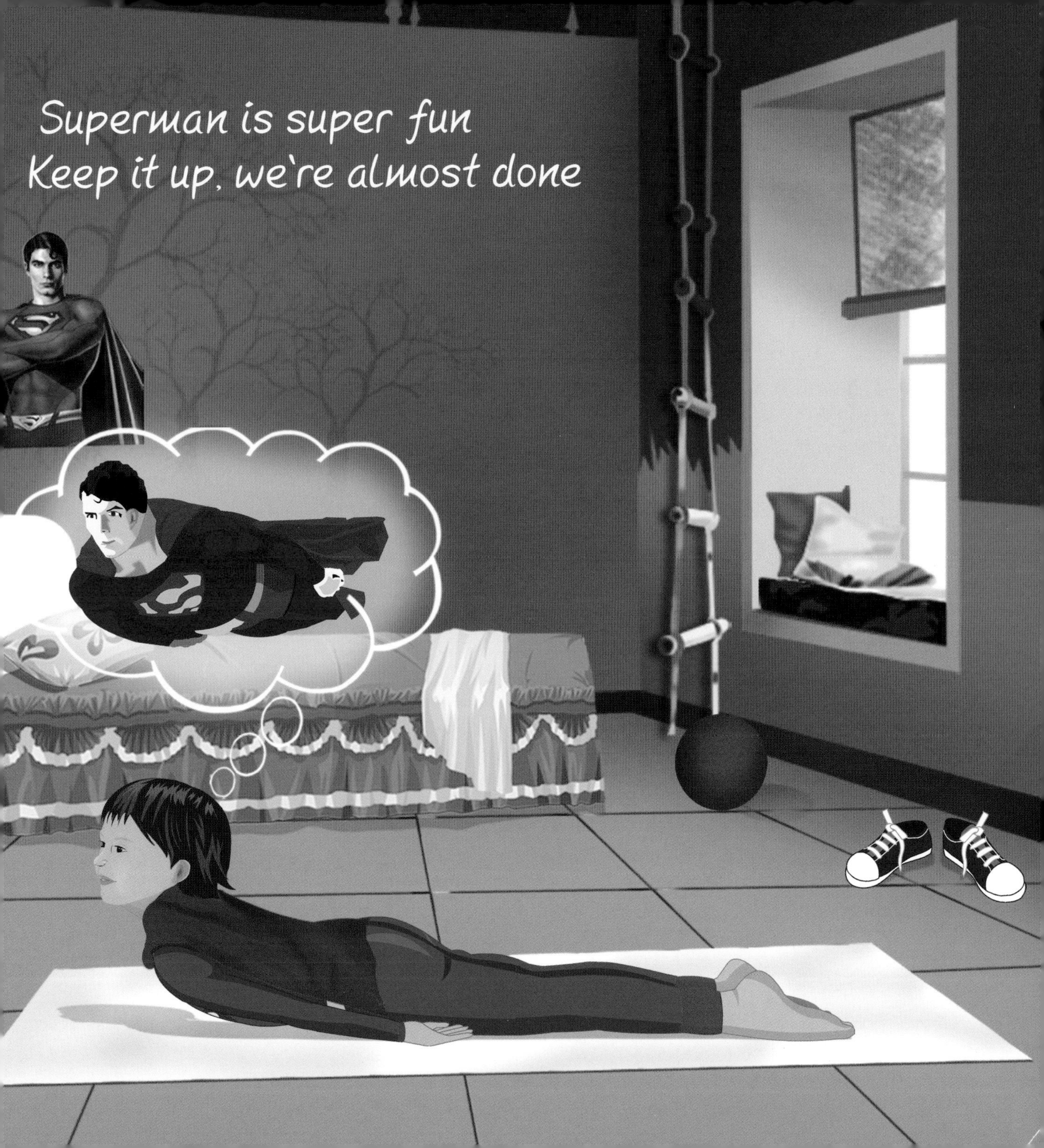
Superman is super fun
Keep it up, we're almost done

Triangle is where you go
To make your energy flow

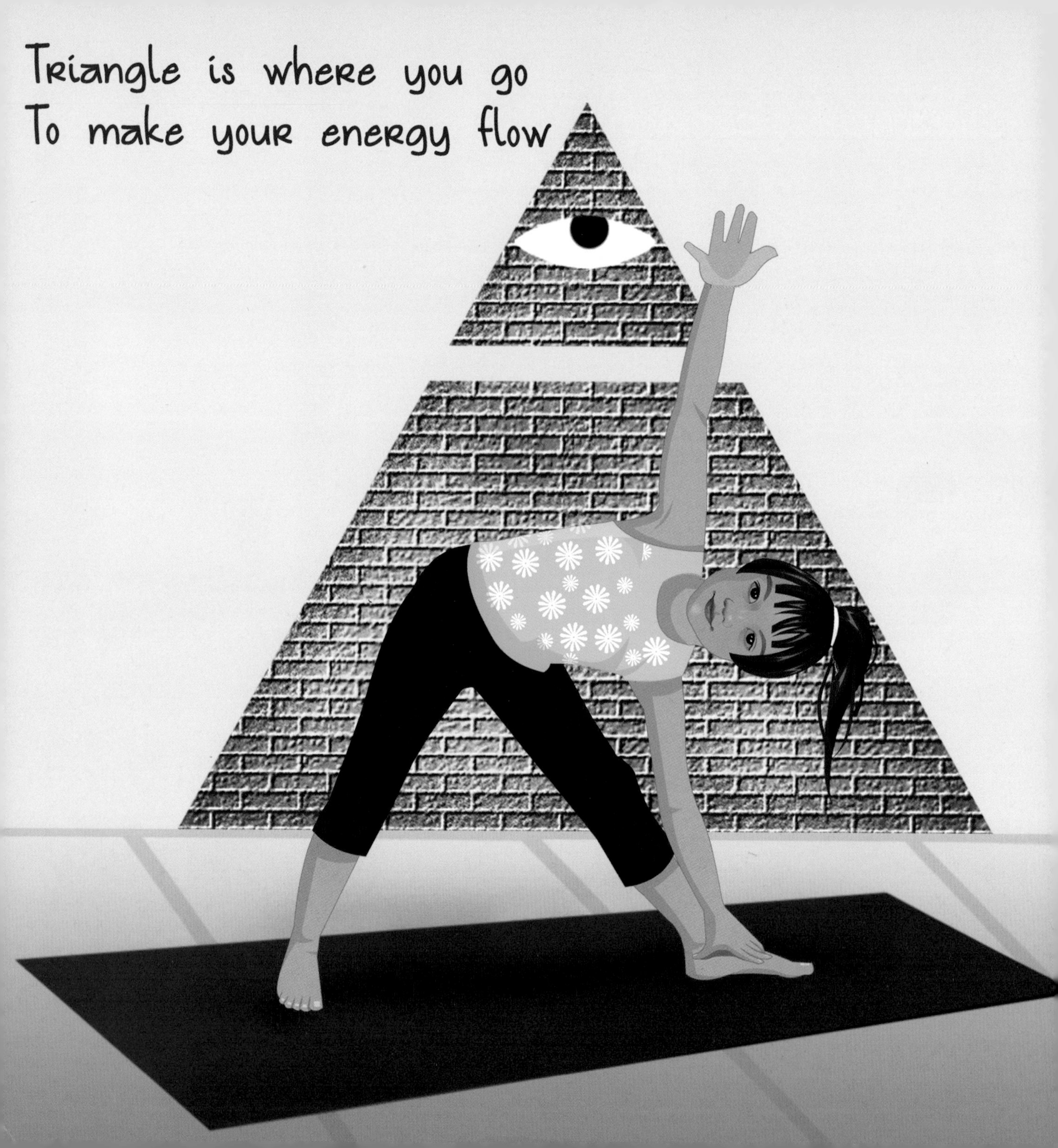

Roll to your back and grab your feet
Happy Baby pose is really neat!

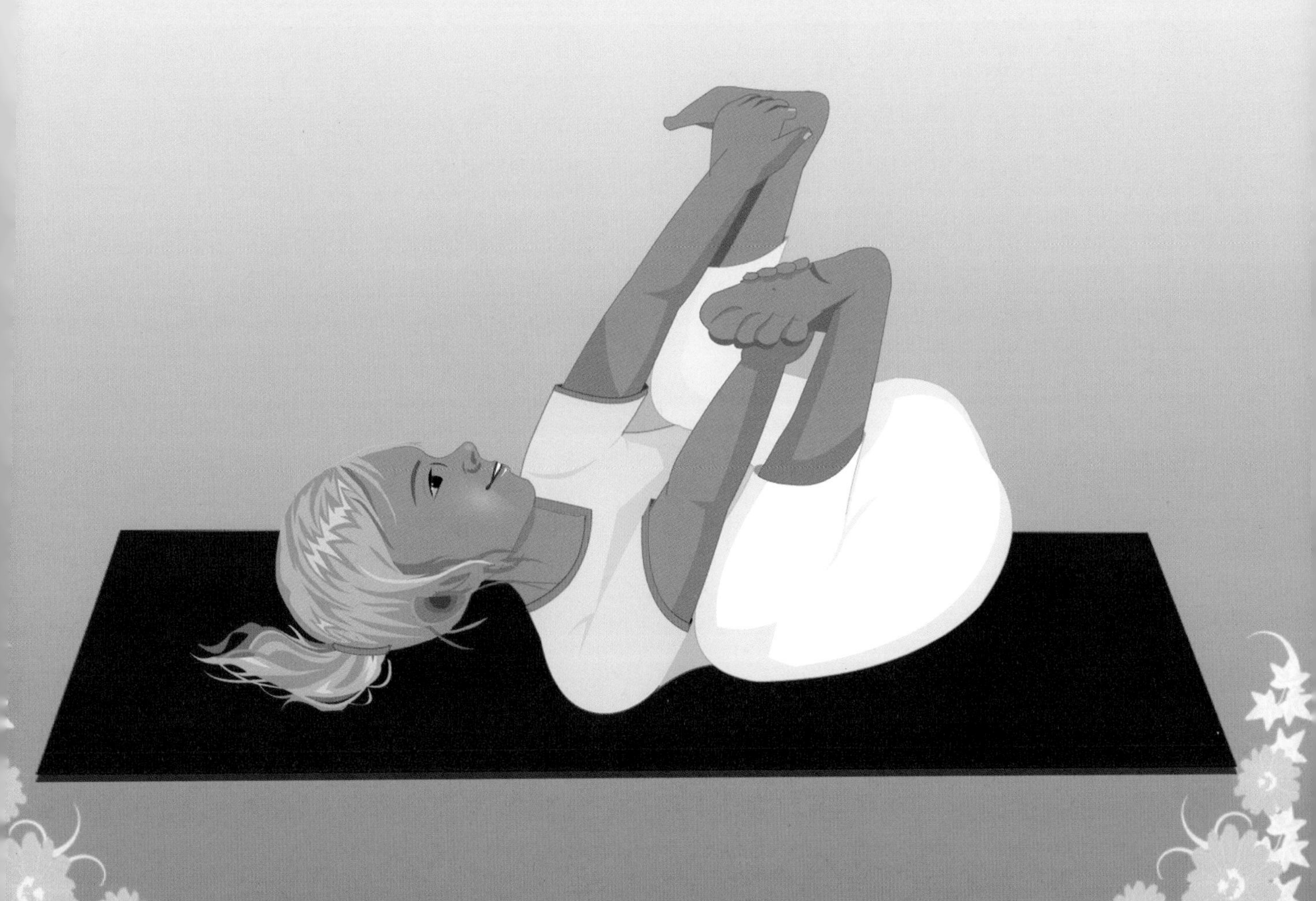

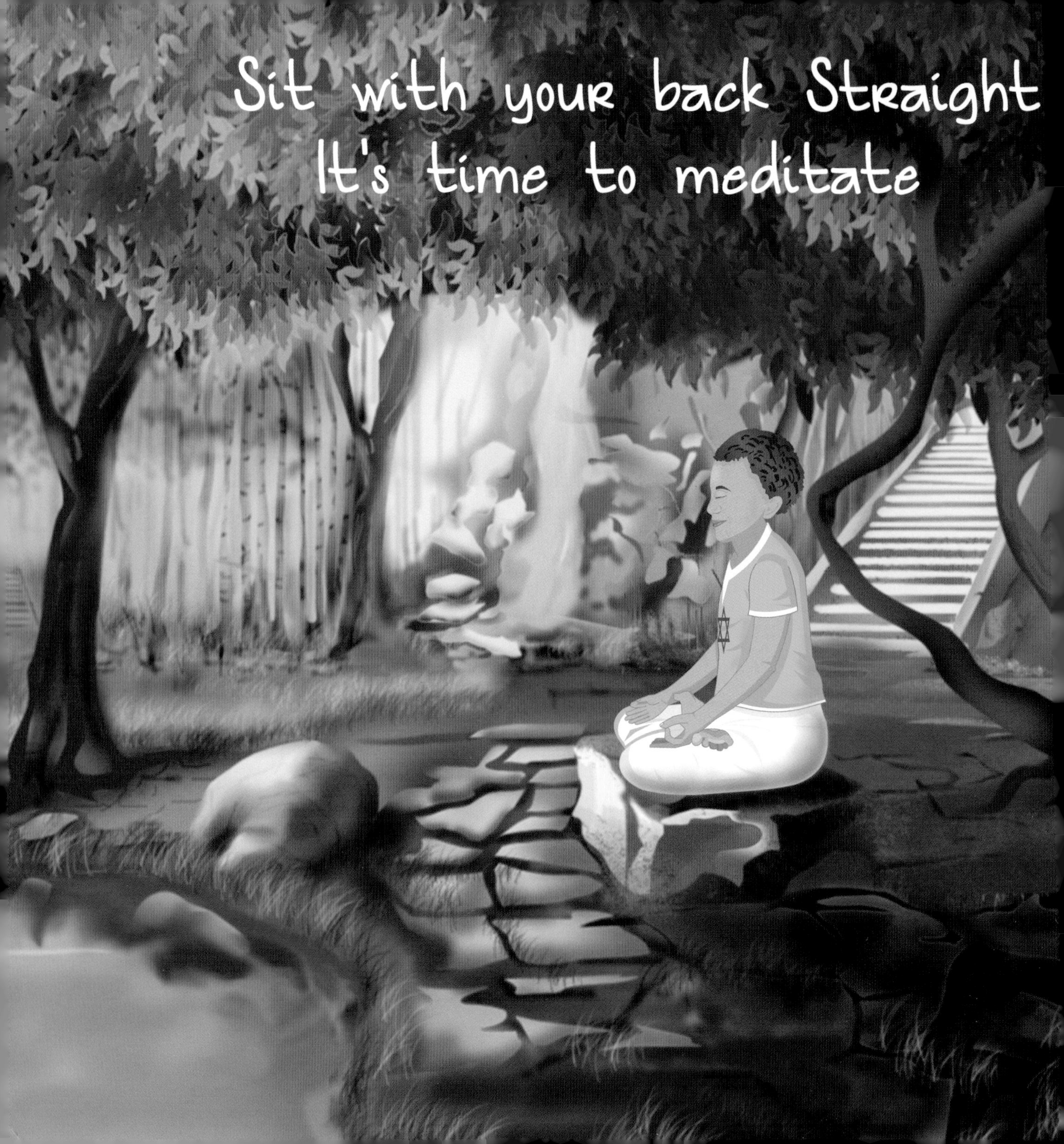
Sit with your back Straight
It's time to meditate

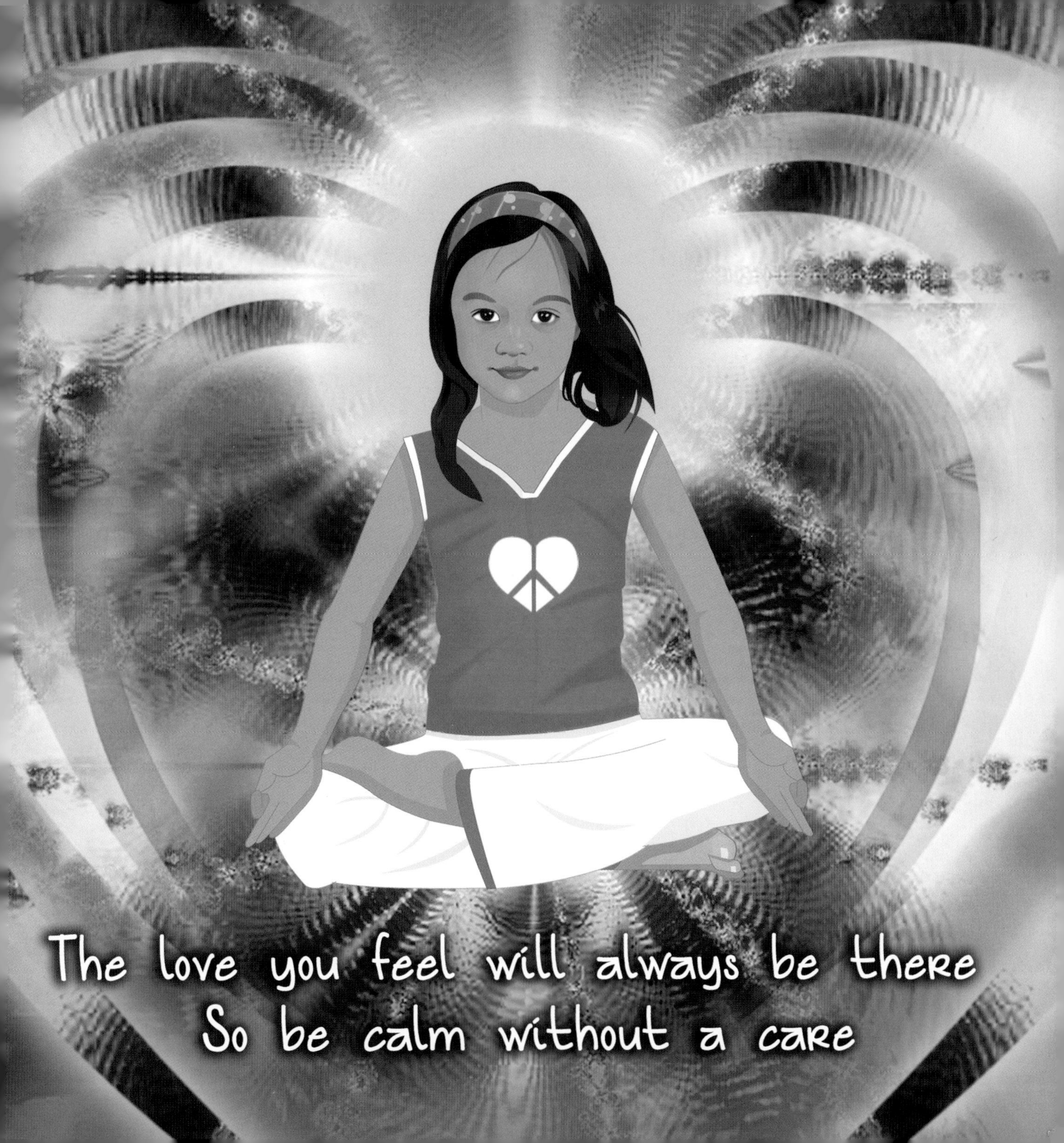
The love you feel will always be there
So be calm without a care

Yoga leaves us Blessed

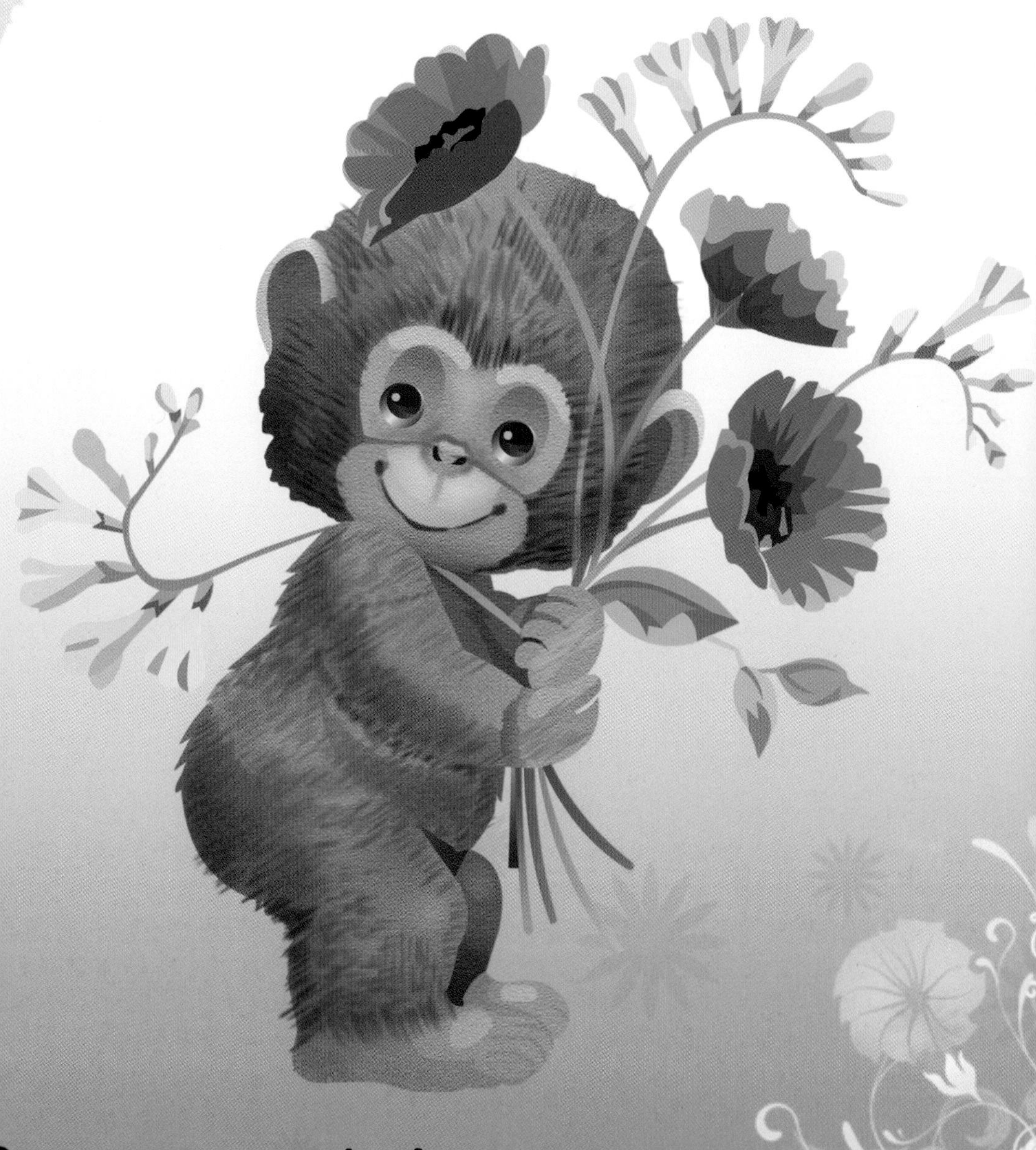

with Grace and Joy...

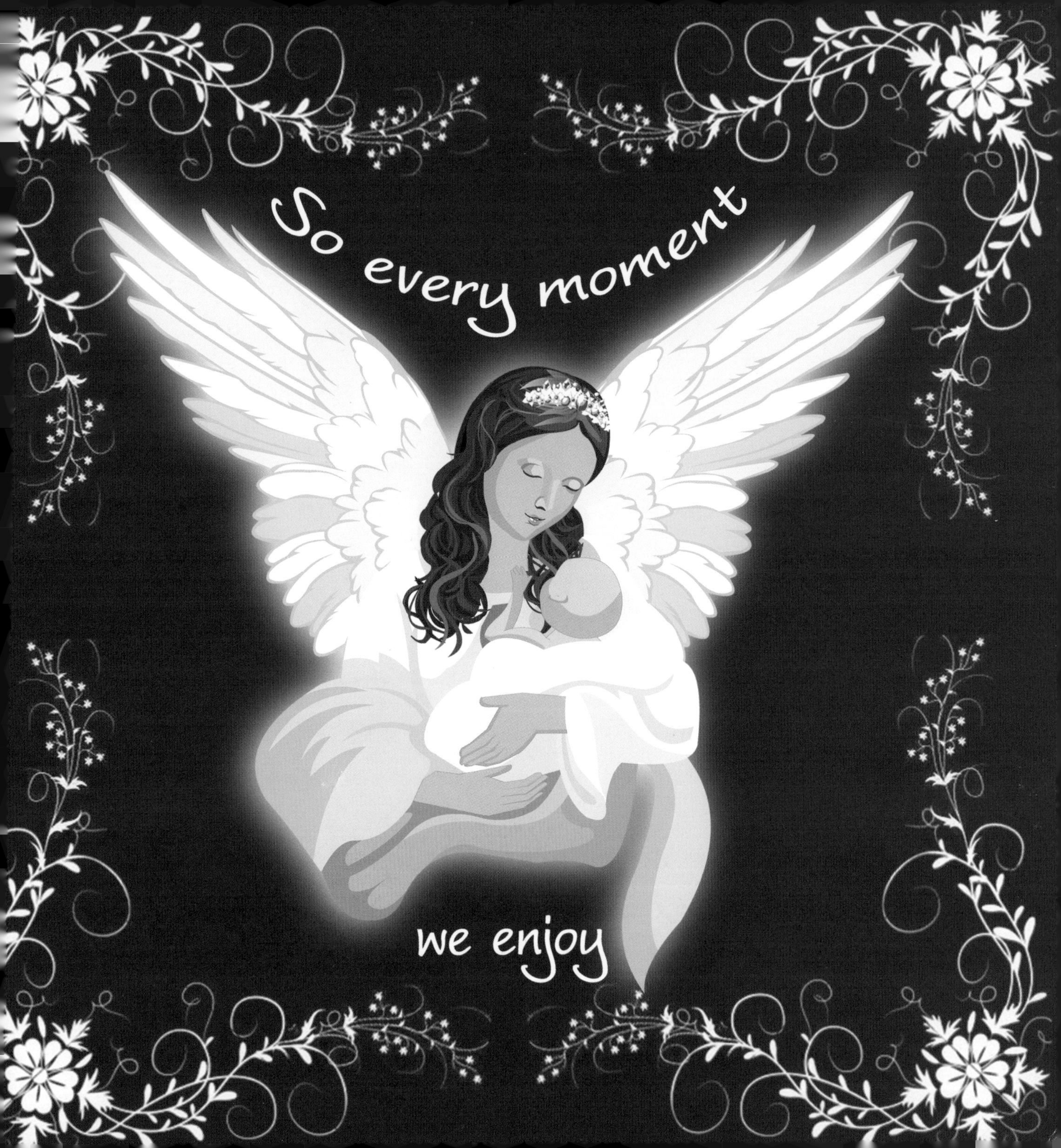
So every moment
we enjoy

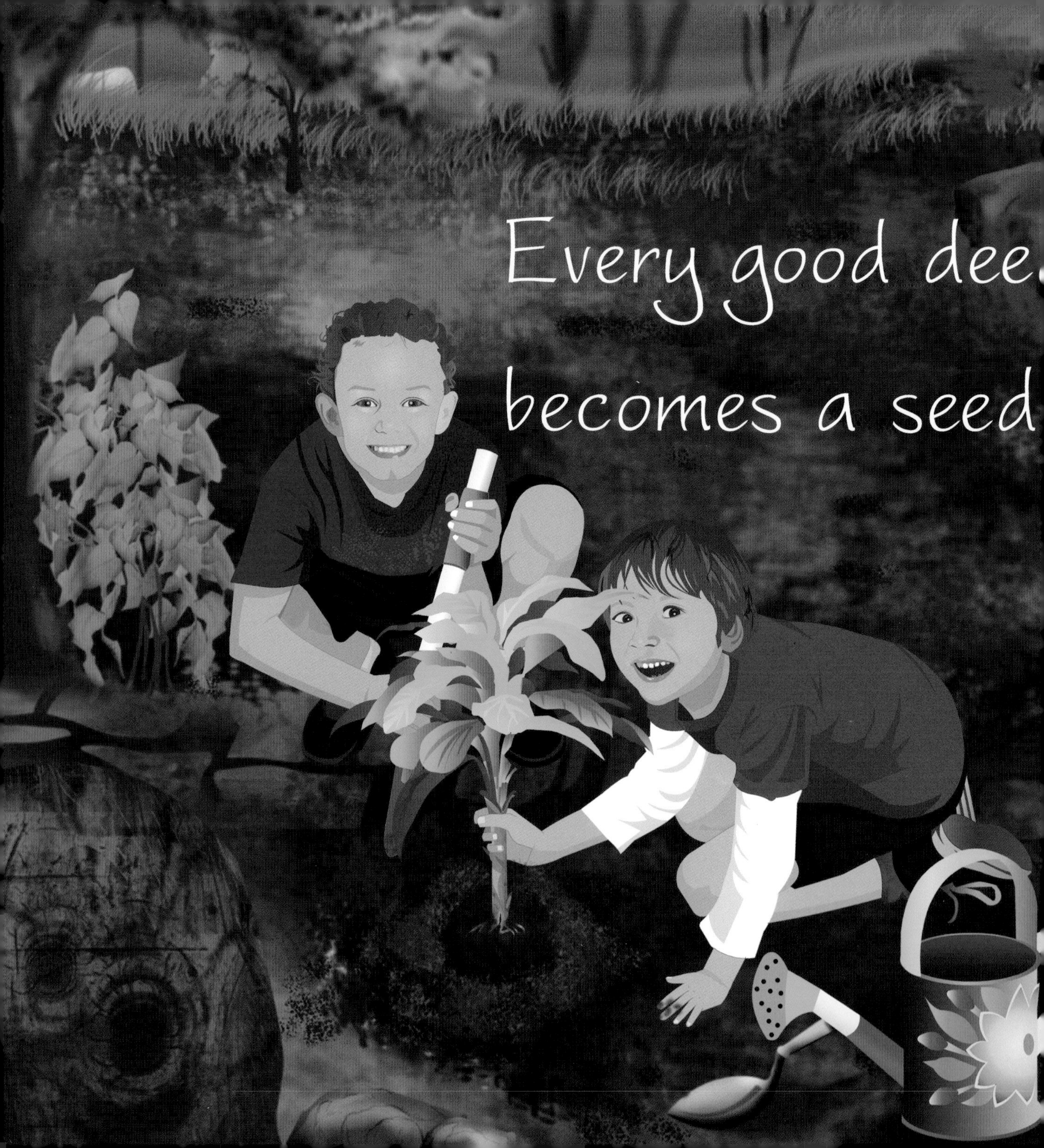
Every good dee
becomes a seed

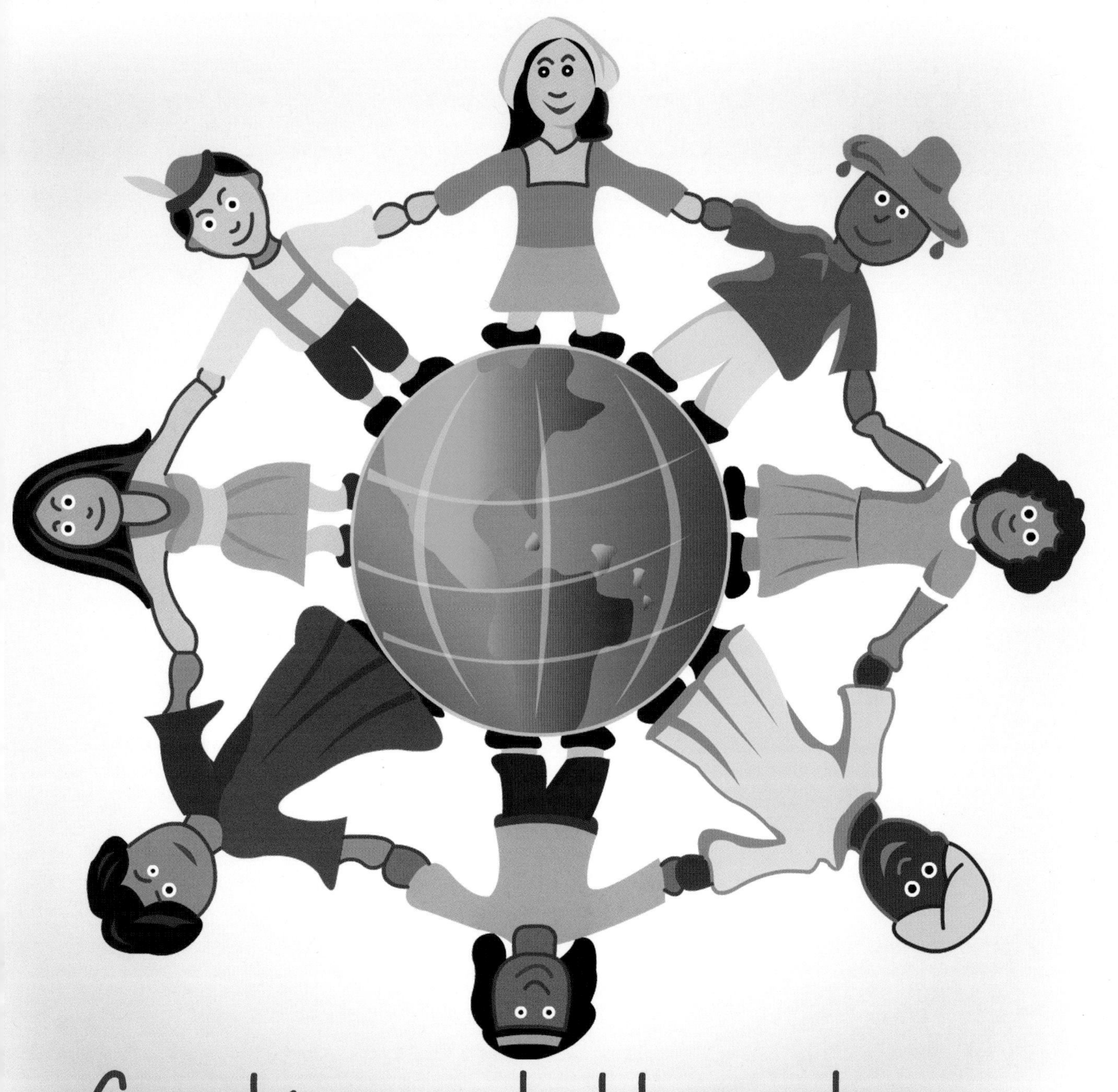

Creating a better place for the whole human race

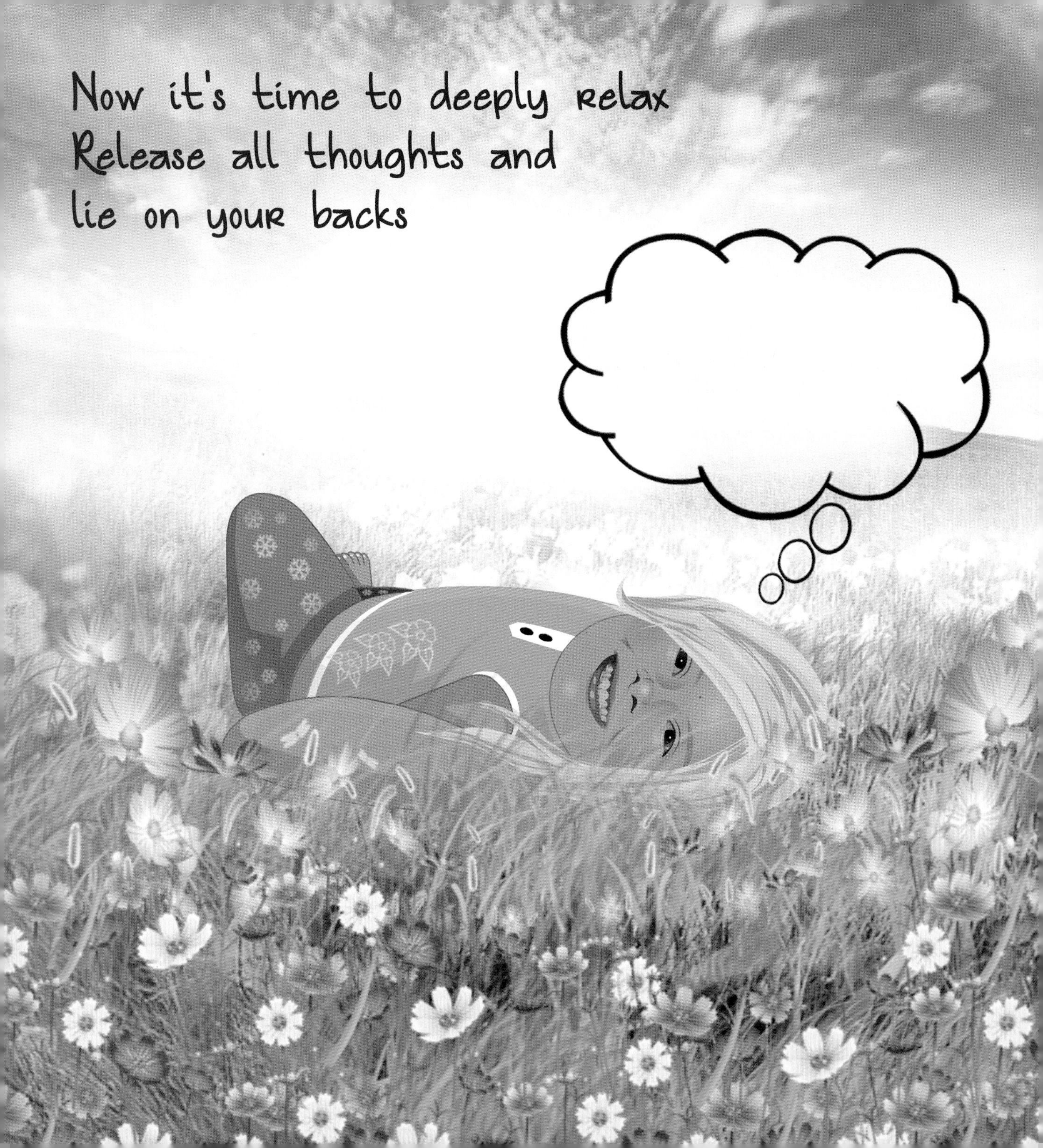
Now it's time to deeply relax
Release all thoughts and
lie on your backs

Remember this deep inner peace
you feel inside
You can feel this way again
whenever you decide

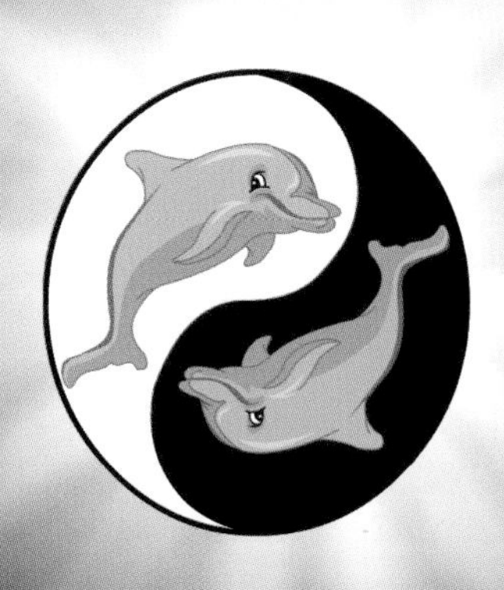

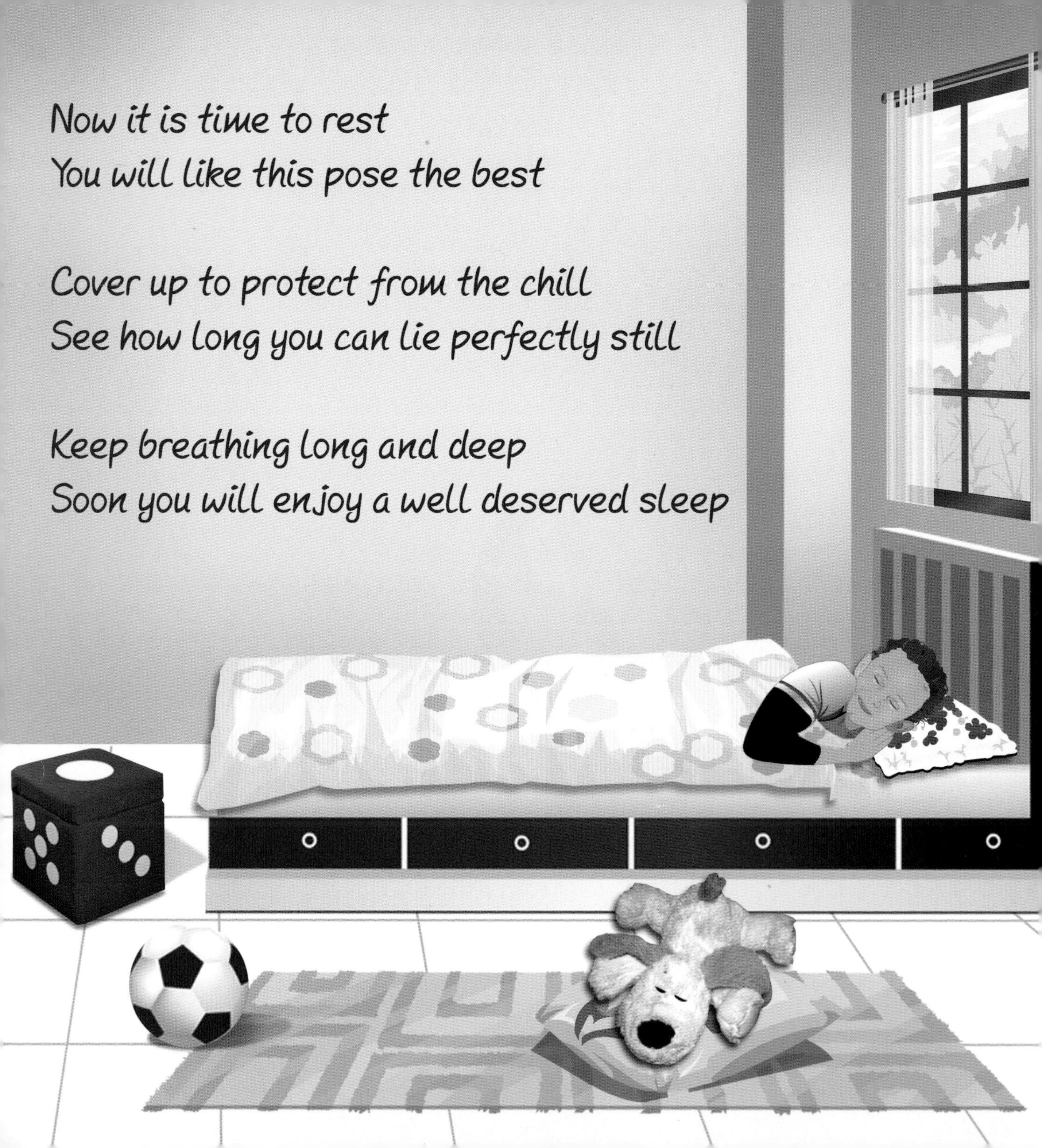

Now it is time to rest
You will like this pose the best

Cover up to protect from the chill
See how long you can lie perfectly still

Keep breathing long and deep
Soon you will enjoy a well deserved sleep